INTERVENTIONAL CARDIOLOGY CLINICS

www.interventional.theclinics.com

Editor-in-Chief

MATTHEW J. PRICE

Renal Disease and Coronary, Peripheral and Structural Interventions

July 2020 • Volume 9 • Number 3

Editor

HITINDER S. GURM

ELSEVIER

1600 John F. Kennedy Boulevard • Suite 1800 • Philadelphia, Pennsylvania, 19103-2899

http://www.theclinics.com

INTERVENTIONAL CARDIOLOGY CLINICS Volume 9, Number 3
July 2020 ISSN 2211-7458, ISBN-13: 978-0-323-76274-8

Editor: Stacy Eastman
Developmental Editor: Donald Mumford

Interventional Cardiology Clinics (ISSN 2211-7458) is published quarterly by Elsevier Inc., 360 Park Avenue South, New York, NY 10010-1710. Months of issue are January, April, July, and October. Subscription prices are USD 209 per year for US individuals, USD 495 for US institutions, USD 100 per year for US students, USD 209 per year for Canadian individuals, USD 590 for Canadian institutions, USD 100 per year for Canadian students, USD 296 per year for international individuals, USD 590 for international institutions, and USD 150 per year for international students. To receive student/resident rate, orders must be accompanied by name of affiliated institution, date of term, and the *signature* of program/residency coordinator on institution letterhead. Orders will be billed at individual rate until proof of status is received. Foreign air speed delivery is included in all *Clinics* subscription prices. All prices are subject to change without notice. **POSTMASTER:** Send address changes to *Interventional Cardiology Clinics*, Elsevier Health Sciences Division, Subscription Customer Service, 3251 Riverport Lane, Maryland Heights, MO 63043. **Customer Service: Telephone: 1-800-654-2452** (U.S. and Canada); **1-314-447-8871** (outside U.S. and Canada). **Fax: 1-314-447-8029. E-mail: journalscustomerservice-usa@elsevier.com (for print support); journalsonlinesupport-usa@elsevier.com (for online support).**

Reprints. For copies of 100 or more of articles in this publication, please contact the Commercial Reprints Department, Elsevier Inc., 360 Park Avenue South, New York, NY 10010-1710. Tel.: 212-633-3874; Fax: 212-633-3820; E-mail: reprints@elsevier.com.

CONTRIBUTORS

EDITOR-IN-CHIEF

MATTHEW J. PRICE, MD
Director, Cardiac Catheterization Laboratory,
Division of Cardiovascular Diseases, Scripps
Clinic, La Jolla, California, USA

EDITOR

HITINDER S. GURM, MD
Professor, Department of Internal Medicine,
Division of Cardiovascular Medicine,
University of Michigan, Frankel Cardiovascular
Center, Ann Arbor, Michigan, USA

AUTHORS

DEVIKA AGGARWAL, MD
Resident, Department of Internal Medicine,
Beaumont Hospital, Royal Oak, Michigan,
USA

LORENZO AZZALINI, MD, PhD, MSc
The Zena and Michael A. Wiener
Cardiovascular Institute, Icahn School of
Medicine at Mount Sinai, New York, New
York, USA

SHWETA BANSAL, MBBS, MD, FASN
Associate Professor of Medicine, Division of
Nephrology, UT Health San Antonio, San
Antonio, Texas, USA

FRANCESCO BELLANDI, MD
Division of Cardiology, Santo Stefano
Hospital, Prato, Italy

CARLO BRIGUORI, MD, PhD
Interventional Cardiology Unit, Mediterranea
Cardiocentro, Naples, Italy

BIMMER CLAESSEN, MD, PhD
The Zena and Michael A. Wiener
Cardiovascular Institute, Icahn School of
Medicine at Mount Sinai, New York, New
York, USA

CARMEN D'AMORE, MD
Interventional Cardiology Unit, Mediterranea
Cardiocentro, Naples, Italy

HITINDER S. GURM, MD
Professor, Department of Internal Medicine,
Division of Cardiovascular Medicine,
University of Michigan, Frankel Cardiovascular
Center, Ann Arbor, Michigan, USA

BADR HARFOUCH, MD, MPH
Division of Cardiology, Department of
Medicine, UT Health San Antonio, San
Antonio, Texas, USA

SANJOG KALRA, MD, MSc
Einstein Heart and Vascular Institute, Einstein
Medical Center Philadelphia, Philadelphia,
Pennsylvania, USA

SAMIR KAPADIA, MD
Chairman, Department of Cardiovascular
Medicine, Cleveland Clinic Foundation,
Cleveland, Ohio, USA

DAVID M. KAYE, MBBS, PhD
Cardiologist, Department of Cardiology,
Alfred Hospital, Department of Medicine,
Nursing and Health Sciences, Monash
University, Head, Heart Failure Research
Group, Baker Heart and Diabetes Institute,
Melbourne, Victoria, Australia

DANIEL KRAUSE, DO
Division of Cardiovascular Medicine, Gill Heart
& Vascular Institute, University of Kentucky,
Lexington, Kentucky, USA

RACHEL G. KROLL
Department of Internal Medicine, Division of
Cardiovascular Medicine, University of
Michigan, Ann Arbor, Michigan, USA

MARIO LEONCINI, MD
Division of Cardiology, Santo Stefano
Hospital, Prato, Italy

SADICHHYA LOHANI, MD
Assistant Professor of Clinical Medicine,
Renal-Electrolyte and Hypertension Division,
Penn Presbyterian Medical Center, Perelman
School of Medicine, University of
Pennsylvania, Philadelphia, Pennsylvania, USA

MAURO MAIOLI, MD
Division of Cardiology, Santo Stefano
Hospital, Prato, Italy

DAMIEN MARYCZ, MD
WakeMed Heart and Vascular, Raleigh, North
Carolina, USA

ROXANA MEHRAN, MD
The Zena and Michael A. Wiener
Cardiovascular Institute, Icahn School of
Medicine at Mount Sinai, New York, New
York, USA

DANIEL S. MENEES, MD
Department of Internal Medicine, Division of
Cardiovascular Medicine, University of
Michigan, Ann Arbor, Michigan, USA

VINAYAK NAGARAJA, MBBS, MS, MMed
(Clin Epi), FRACP
Department of Cardiovascular Medicine,
Cleveland Clinic Foundation, Cleveland, Ohio,
USA

SHANE NANAYAKKARA, MBBS, PhD
Cardiologist, Department of Cardiology,
Alfred Hospital, Research Fellow, Baker Heart
and Diabetes Institute, Department of
Medicine, Nursing and Health Sciences,
Monash University, Melbourne, Victoria,
Australia

JOHNY NICOLAS, MD
The Zena and Michael A. Wiener
Cardiovascular Institute, Icahn School of
Medicine at Mount Sinai, New York, New
York, USA

SILVIA NUZZO, PhD
IRCCS, SDN, Naples, Italy

RAHUL N. PATEL, MD
Nephrology Fellow, Division of Nephrology,
UT Health San Antonio, San Antonio, Texas,
USA

ANAND PRASAD, MD, FACC, FSCAI
Division of Cardiology, Department of
Medicine, UT Health San Antonio, San
Antonio, Texas, USA

MICHAEL R. RUDNICK, MD
Associate Professor of Medicine, Renal-
Electrolyte and Hypertension Division, Penn
Presbyterian Medical Center, Perelman School
of Medicine, University of Pennsylvania,
Philadelphia, Pennsylvania, USA

RICHARD SOLOMON, MD, FACP, FASN
Director, Division of Nephrology, Patrick
Professor of Medicine, The Robert Larner,
M.D. College of Medicine, University of
Vermont, University of Vermont Medical
Center, Burlington, Vermont, USA

NADIA R. SUTTON, MD, MPH
Department of Internal Medicine, Division of
Cardiovascular Medicine, University of
Michigan, Ann Arbor, Michigan, USA

ANNA TOSO, MD
Division of Cardiology, Santo Stefano
Hospital, Prato, Italy

PRASANTHI YELAVARTHY, MD
Department of Internal Medicine, Division of
Cardiovascular Medicine, University of
Michigan, Ann Arbor, Michigan, USA

KHALED M. ZIADA, MD, FACC, FSCAI
Director, Interventional Services, Director,
Cardiovascular Interventional Fellowship
Program, Clinical Chief of Cardiology, Division
of Cardiovascular Medicine, Gill Heart &
Vascular Institute, University of Kentucky,
Lexington, Kentucky, USA

CONTENTS

Cardiovascular and renal diseases share common pathophysiological grounds, risk factors, and therapies. The 2 entities are closely interlinked and often coexist. The prevalence of kidney disease among cardiac patients is increasing. Patients have an atypical clinical presentation and variable disease manifestation versus the general population. Renal impairment limits therapeutic options and worsens prognosis. Meticulous treatment and close monitoring are required to ensure safety and avoid deterioration of kidney and heart functions. This review highlights recent advances in the diagnosis and treatment of cardiac pathologies, including coronary artery disease, arrhythmia, and heart failure, in patients with decreased renal function.

History of contrast dates back to the 1890s, with the invention of the radiograph. Nephrotoxicity has been a main limitation in ideal contrast media (CM). High-osmolar contrast media no longer are in clinical use due to overwhelming evidence supporting greater nephrotoxicity with these CM compared with current CM. Contrast-induced nephropathy (CIN) remains a common cause of in-hospital acute kidney injury. The choice contrast agent is determined mainly by cost and institution practice. This review focuses on the history, chemical properties, and experimental and clinical studies on the various groups of CM and their role in CIN.

Passing contrast media through the renal vascular bed leads to vasoconstriction. The perfusion decrease leads to ischemia of tubular cells. Through ischemia and direct toxicity to renal tubular cells, reactive oxygen species formation is increased, enhancing the effect of vasoconstrictive mediators and decreasing the bioavailability of vasodilative mediators. Reactive oxygen species formation leads to oxidative damage to tubular cells. These interacting pathways lead to tubular necrosis. In the pathophysiology of contrast-induced acute kidney injury, low osmolar and iso-osmolar agents have theoretic advantages and disadvantages; however, clinically the difference in incidence of contrast-induced acute kidney injury has not changed.

Contrast-induced acute kidney injury (CI-AKI) is the acute onset of renal injury following exposure to iodinated contrast media. Several definitions have been used, which complicates the estimation of the epidemiological relevance of this condition and comparisons in outcome research. The incidence of CI-AKI increases as a function of patient and procedure complexity in coronary, endovascular, and structural interventions. CI-AKI is associated with a high burden of short- and long-term adverse events, and leads to increased healthcare costs. This review will provide an overview of the definitions, epidemiology, and implications of CI-AKI in patients undergoing coronary, endovascular, and structural catheter-based procedures.

Injection of contrast media is the foundation of invasive and interventional cardiovascular practice. Iodine-based contrast was first used in the 1920s for urologic procedures and examinations. The initially used agents had high ionic and osmolar concentrations, which led to significant side effects, namely nausea, vomiting, and hypotension. Newer contrast agents had lower ionic concentrations and lower osmolarity. Modifications to the ionic structure and iodine content led to the development of ionic low-osmolar, nonionic low-osmolar, and nonionic iso-osmolar contrast media. Contemporary contrast agents are better tolerated and produce fewer major side effects.

Chronic kidney disease is a major risk factor for developing coronary artery disease, serving as an independent risk factor while overlapping with other risk factors. Percutaneous coronary intervention is a cornerstone of therapy for coronary artery disease and requires contrast media, which can contribute to renal injury. Identifying patients at risk for contrast-induced nephropathy is critical for preventing renal injury, which is associated with short- and long-term mortality. Determination of the potential risk for contrast-induced nephropathy and a new need for dialysis using validated risk prediction tools is a method of identifying patients at high risk for this complication.

Contrast-induced acute kidney injury (CI-AKI) is a common complication after intravascular injection of iodinated contrast media, and it is associated with a prolonged in-hospital stay and unfavorable outcome. CI-AKI occurs in 5% to 20% among hospitalized patients. Its diagnosis relies on the increase in serum creatinine levels, which is a late biomarker of kidney injury. Novel and early serum and urinary biomarkers have been identified to detect kidney damage before the expected serum creatinine increase.

Since the first peripheral endovascular intervention (PVI) in 1964, the procedure's technical aspects and indications have advanced significantly. Today, endovascular procedures span the spectrum of presentations from acute limb ischemia to critical limb ischemia and symptomatic limiting claudication. Goals of PVI remain restoring limb perfusion, minimizing rates of amputation and mortality, and sparing the need for the high-risk bypass surgery. Unfortunately, there are no large randomized controlled trials that address the optimal approach to peripheral arterial disease revascularization in chronic kidney disease (CKD) patients.

Chronic kidney disease patients have a high prevalence of severe valvular heart disease, which reduces life expectancy. Transcatheter valve interventions has revamped the way we manage severe valvular heart disease and are an attractive alternative to invasive surgery in patients with chronic kidney disease and severe valvular heart disease. This review summarizes the impact of transcatheter valve interventions in patients with severe valvular heart disease and chronic kidney disease.

Different pharmacologic agents have been tested in the effort to prevent contrast-induced acute kidney injury (AKI) in the last two decades. To date, however, no individual drug has received unanimous approval for this aim. Since 2014 statins have been included as preventive treatment in the European guidelines for revascularization procedures in cardiac patients. The present update presents the latest findings in this field focusing on the changing paradigms in the definition and consequently the approach to nephroprotection that considers clinical prognosis as the major issue. We note the current shift from attention to contrast-induced AKI to contrast-associated AKI.

The literature (in English) was accessed to review the evidence that administration of fluids is protective of contrast-associated acute kidney injury (CA-AKI). The evidence was evaluated with the intent of understanding mechanisms of protection. Prospective randomized trials comparing oral versus intravenous fluid, sodium chloride versus no intravenous fluid, sodium bicarbonate versus sodium chloride, and forced matched hydration versus intravenous sodium chloride provided the data. In general, the more fluid administered, the lower the incidence of CA-AKI. However, understanding the mechanism of this beneficial effect suggests that it is the urine output that most directly affects the incidence of CA-AKI.

Contrast-induced acute kidney injury is not uncommon after percutaneous coronary intervention, particularly in high-risk patients. Pharmacologic approaches have not demonstrated significant benefit, and numerous device-based approaches exist targeting a variety of pathways. In this review, we summarize the most recent interventions and the evidence behind them.

Contrast-induced acute kidney injury is a common complication in patients undergoing invasive procedures and is associated with increased mortality and morbidity. There is no effective approach to the management of this complication, and prevention remains of paramount importance. The 3 pillars of prevention are identification of high-risk patients, appropriate hydration before and after contrast exposure, eGFR-based contrast dosing and use of ultra-low contrast volume in high-risk patients. Most evidence supporting these practices is derived from patients undergoing coronary angiography or percutaneous coronary intervention but these basic principles can be applied to most patients undergoing contrast-based procedures in the catheterization laboratory.

RENAL DISEASE AND CORONARY, PERIPHERAL AND STRUCTURAL INTERVENTIONS

THE CLINICS ARE NOW AVAILABLE ONLINE!

Access your subscription at:
www.theclinics.com

PREFACE

Renal Disease and Coronary, Peripheral and Structural Interventions

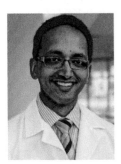

Hitinder S. Gurm, MD
Editor

Interventional cardiology sits at an important intersection of renal and cardiac disease. Patients with cardiovascular disease are more prone to develop renal disease, while those with renal disease are at a greater risk of developing cardiac disease. Patients with chronic kidney disease commonly need to undergo cardiovascular interventions and are at a higher risk of both renal and nonrenal complications. Acute kidney injury (AKI) in patients undergoing cardiovascular procedures is associated with increased mortality, morbidity, and health care expense. There is no effective treatment for AKI, and accordingly, there is considerable interest in understanding and preventing this common complication. Since the last issue of *Interventional Cardiology Clinics* dedicated to "Renal Complications in the Catheterization Laboratory" was published in 2014, there have been multiple high-impact studies on the subject that have provided much needed clarity to this field. Interventional cardiologists have been at the forefront of these efforts and have been exploring novel innovations and device-based strategies to reduce the risk of AKI, and to better treat patients with chronic kidney disease. It is our privilege to present to you an issue of *Interventional Cardiology Clinics* that provides a comprehensive, yet practical overview of the juncture of renal disease and the catheterization laboratory. The authors are internationally recognized experts in the field of cardiorenal medicine and readily volunteered their knowledge and time to create an outstanding review of this complex subject. In the initial reviews, they discuss the epidemiology and implications of renal disease in patients with cardiovascular disease, and those undergoing structural and peripheral interventions. Subsequent articles are devoted to prediction and pathophysiology of contrast-induced AKI. Additional articles cover the use of diagnostic biomarkers, differences in nephrotoxicity between contrast agents, the comparative effectiveness of different

Intervent Cardiol Clin 9 (2020) xi–xii
https://doi.org/10.1016/j.iccl.2020.04.001
2211-7458/20/© 2020 Published by Elsevier Inc.

hydration strategies, and other device and pharmacologic preventive measures. One article is dedicated to nonrenal complications of iodinated contrast media: even though infrequent, these can be associated with severe consequences, and every interventional cardiologist and catheterization laboratory needs to understand and be able to prevent and treat them.

I would again like to thank all the authors who graciously accepted our invitation to contribute to this issue of *Interventional Cardiology Clinics*. We hope you find the updated perspective in this issue informative, and useful in your daily practice.

Hitinder S. Gurm, MD
Division of Cardiovascular Medicine
Department of Internal Medicine
Frankel Cardiovascular Center
2A 192F, 1500 East Medical Center Drive
Ann Arbor, MI 48109-5853, USA

E-mail address:
hgurm@med.umich.edu

Implications of Kidney Disease in the Cardiac Patient

Johny Nicolas, MD, Bimmer Claessen, MD, PhD,
Roxana Mehran, MD*

KEYWORDS

- Chronic kidney disease • Cardiovascular disease • Chronic renal failure • Heart failure
- Coronary artery disease • Renal disease • CKD

KEY POINTS

- A large proportion of cardiac patients have renal disease that impacts prognosis and narrow down therapeutic options.
- Invasive and noninvasive therapies for coronary artery disease exhibit adverse toxic effects on the kidneys.
- Renal disease often co-occurs with atrial fibrillation and requires meticulous choice of anticoagulants and close monitoring of adverse effects.
- Recent and ongoing studies investigating novel heart failure therapies show promise in patients with decreased kidney function.
- Additional prospective studies focusing on the diagnosis and management of cardiovascular diseases in patients with renal impairment are needed.

INTRODUCTION

The increasing prevalence of hypertension and obesity in developed countries is a central driver of the twenty-first century's epidemic of cardiovascular diseases.[1] Cardiac patients often present with concomitant renal pathologies that worsen prognosis and limit therapeutic options. The 2 organs are tightly linked and failure of either leads to dysfunction of the other in a vicious cycle.[2] The heart–kidney relationship was first elucidated in nineteenth century by Richard Bright, a pioneer researcher in renal diseases, who described structural changes in cardiac tissue biopsies of patients with chronic kidney disease (CKD).[3] Based on these findings and additional evidence revealing common pathophysiologic grounds between the 2 entities, the concept of cardio-renal syndrome had been established.[4,5] Indeed, over the past years, it has become more evident that the epidemiology, risk factors, prevention, and treatment of renal and cardiac diseases are interrelated and closely dependent.[6]

Cardiovascular diseases manifest clinically in several forms, including but not limited to coronary artery disease (CAD), cardiac arrhythmias, and heart failure. In contrast, kidney disease encompasses vascular, glomerular, and tubular pathologies that lead to a progressive decrease in the glomerular filtration rate (GFR) to less than 60 mL/min/1.73 m^2 and disturbances in electrolytes and plasma proteins. The proportion of elderly living with cardiovascular disease is increasing owing to major improvements in cardiovascular care. Nonetheless, as age advances the number of comorbidities increases and impacts disease progression. This review discusses how worsening renal function dictates the choice of both invasive and noninvasive interventions

The Zena and Michael A. Wiener Cardiovascular Institute, Icahn School of Medicine at Mount Sinai, One Gustave L. Levy Place, Box 1030, New York, NY 10029-6574, USA
* Corresponding author.
E-mail address: roxana.mehran@mountsinai.org

Intervent Cardiol Clin 9 (2020) 265–278
https://doi.org/10.1016/j.iccl.2020.03.002

and affects prognosis in patients with cardiac disease.

CORONARY ARTERY DISEASE AND RENAL IMPAIRMENT

CKD is a well-established risk factor for CAD.[7–9] It often coexists with other traditional and uremia-related cardiovascular risk factors that worsen prognosis (Fig. 1).[10–13] Indeed, the probability of developing CAD increases linearly as the GFR decreases below 90 mL/min/1.73 m^2 and doubles with disease progression especially when GFR falls below 60 mL/min/1.73 m^2.[14]

The Underlying Pathophysiology

The existence of renal impairment on top of cardiac disease is by itself a major risk factor that accelerates atherosclerosis through a sequelae of reactions: monocytes recruitment followed by ingression and conversion to macrophages and foam cells, breakdown of elastic lamina, and development of atheroma that obstructs the lumen of vessels through invasion of the adventitia.[15] Indeed, calcification of the media and subintima layers in large vessels increases with worsening kidney function and is highly correlated with mortality in end-stage renal disease.[16] Autopsy studies of atherosclerotic plaques in patients with CKD showed quantitative similarities, but qualitative differences in terms of calcification and an abundance of calcium hydroxyapatite crystals deposited in the extracellular matrix.[17–19] The exact mechanism by which increased calcification occurs is not well-understood, but is probably related to inflammatory reactions that increase oxidative stress in atherosclerotic plaques of patients with

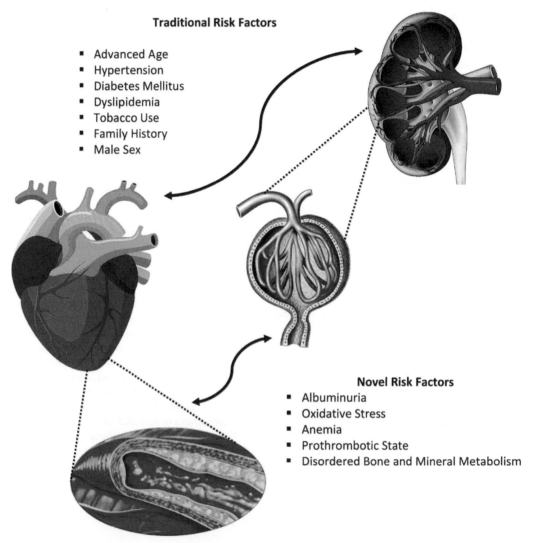

Traditional Risk Factors

- Advanced Age
- Hypertension
- Diabetes Mellitus
- Dyslipidemia
- Tobacco Use
- Family History
- Male Sex

Novel Risk Factors

- Albuminuria
- Oxidative Stress
- Anemia
- Prothrombotic State
- Disordered Bone and Mineral Metabolism

Fig. 1. CAD traditional and novel risk factors in patients with renal impairment.

CKD.[20] In addition, loss of phosphorus hemostasis owing to decreased renal excretion results in hyperphosphatemia and increased stimulation of vascular smooth muscle cells to undergo osteoblastic changes. In addition, carbamylation of lipoprotein residues in low-density lipoprotein (LDL) cholesterol accelerates the progression of atherosclerotic disease in CKD.[21] In fact, the Clinical Outcomes Utilizing Revascularization and Drug Evaluation (COURAGE, NCT00007657) trial in addition to multiple registries showed that the prevalence of triple vessel disease and left main disease as seen on angiography among patients with CKD was higher than in patients without CKD.[22,23]

Clinical Presentation

The majority of patients with CKD do not experience typical symptoms of acute myocardial infarction (MI) such as chest, shoulder, or jaw pain. Instead, dyspnea is the most frequently reported chief complaint in the emergency room.[24] Moreover, the clinical presentation is largely dependent on the level of renal function decline; patients with advanced disease have the least typical symptoms, whereas patients with early-stage disease often present with a picture similar to the general population.[25] Furthermore, dialysis-dependent patients often have recurrent hemodialysis-induced ischemic cardiac injury. This process is commonly known as myocardial stunning, which is associated with an intradialytic drop in blood pressure, long-term loss of systolic function, and an increase in cardiovascular events and mortality rates.[26,27] Indeed, most of these patients have limited mobility and thus have minimal expression of exercise-induced chest pain. Consequently, clinicians should have a lower threshold for suspicion of ischemic heart disease in this particular population.

Diagnosis

Conventional tools used in the diagnosis of CAD are often less reliable in patients with renal disease. Owing to electrolyte disturbances, nonspecific abnormalities are frequently encountered on the electrocardiogram of patients with CKD.[28,29] Hence, the electrocardiogram is often not reliable and other diagnostic modalities are used to support the diagnosis of acute coronary syndromes. However, even more advanced techniques such as stress test and pharmacologic perfusion imaging show high rates of false-negative and false-positive results in patients with renal impairment.[30] Indeed, a meta-analysis examining the performance of cardiac stress testing showed that, in potential kidney transplant candidates, dobutamine stress echocardiography and myocardial perfusion scintigraphy had a sensitivity of 80% and 69% and a specificity of 89% and 80%, respectively.[31] Moreover, patients with CKD are frequently unable to reach diagnostic workloads during stress testing owing to limited physical activity.[32] In addition, the ability to detect ST-segment changes during exercise is often limited by left ventricular hypertrophy, altered baseline coronary flow reserve, ischemic balance in multivessel disease, and large interobserver variability in interpretation of the results.

Treatment Modalities

Lipid-lowering therapy

The management of CAD in patients with renal impairment is challenging. These patients are often under-represented in large studies and evidence supporting various recommendations is weak.[33] Lipid-lowering therapy, a main pillar of CAD medical management, is controversial among patients with CKD because the cardiovascular benefits of statins seen in the general population shrink with decreasing renal function and are almost abolished in dialysis-dependent patients.[34,35] The 2018 American College of Cardiology/American Heart Association guidelines on management of blood cholesterol recommend (Class IIa, Level B-R) the initiation of moderate-intensity statin (with or without ezetimibe) in adults with CKD but not needing dialysis and LDL cholesterol level of 70 to 189 mg/dL or greater along with a 10-year atherosclerotic cardiovascular disease) risk of 7.5% or greater.[36] Conversely, in patients with advanced kidney disease requiring dialysis, the initiation of statins is not recommended (Grade III, Level B-R).

Other than statins, PCSK-9 inhibitors are currently being tested as a potential antidyslipidemia drug in patients with CKD. In a substudy of the Further Cardiovascular Outcomes Research with PCSK9 Inhibition in Subjects with Elevated Risk (FOURIER) trial, patients with CKD with clinically evident atherosclerosis, LDL cholesterol of 70 mg/dL or greater, and receiving statins were randomized to either evolocumab or placebo and followed for 48 weeks.[37] As compared with the placebo group, a decrease in LDL cholesterol from baseline was similar across CKD groups: 59% (preserved kidney function), 59% (stage 2 CKD), and 58% (stage 3 CKD or higher).[37] Moreover, the relative clinical efficacy and safety of evolocumab were consistent across the 3 groups. Interestingly, the absolute decrease in a secondary end point (a composite of cardiovascular death, MI, or stroke) was numerically greater in advanced stage CKD (−2.5% in stage 3 CKD or higher vs −1.7% in preserved renal function).[37]

Revascularization or optimal medical therapy alone?

The choice of optimal CAD therapy is controversial in patients with impaired kidney function. A systematic review of 5 randomized trials including patients with CKD (n = 1453) who presented with unstable angina or non–ST-segment elevation MI showed that an early invasive strategy is superior to a conservative one in decreasing the risk of death, nonfatal reinfarction, and rehospitalization.[38] Yet, a report from the National Cardiovascular Data Acute Coronary Treatment and Intervention Outcomes Network registry revealed that patients with moderate to severe CKD presenting with acute coronary syndromes are less likely to receive evidence-based therapies (beta-blockers, aspirin, clopidogrel, etc) or to undergo revascularization as compared with patients with normal kidney function.[39]

In major trials comparing invasive and conservative strategies for the management of stable ischemic heart disease, patients with CKD were either excluded or underrepresented. The International Study of Comparative Health Effectiveness with Medical and Invasive Approaches-Chronic Kidney Disease study (ISCHEMIA-CKD; NCT01985360) is a large randomized trial comparing routine invasive therapy (percutaneous coronary intervention [PCI] or coronary artery bypass grafting [CABG]) to optimal medical therapy in stable patients with moderate to severe ischemia and CKD. The primary outcome of interest, death or MI, occurred in 36.7% of patients on medical therapy and 36.4% of those who underwent invasive procedures at 2.3 years of follow-up (invasive/medical therapy, hazard ratio [HR], 0.70; 95% confidence interval [CI], 0.46–1.05 for severe ischemia; and invasive/medical therapy, HR, 1.30; 95% CI, 0.94–1.79 for moderate ischemia; $P_{interaction}$ = .02).[40] Consequently, the ISCHEMIA-CKD investigators concluded that invasive therapy does not lead to a decrease in death and MI as compared with medical therapy in patients with CKD with stable ischemic heart disease.

Percutaneous coronary intervention or coronary artery bypass grafting?

Both PCI and CABG carry an increased risk for periprocedural complications in patients with CKD as compared with the general population.

Despite several observational studies showing survival benefits with revascularization compared with medical therapy, patients with CKD are less likely to undergo either procedure than those with preserved renal function.[41–43] In addition, large-scale registries showed favorable short- and long-term outcomes with early revascularization in patients with CKD presenting with acute coronary syndromes.[44,45] Nonetheless, patients with renal impairment are often underrepresented in or even excluded from randomized trials comparing the 2 techniques. Hence, evidence supporting the use of one intervention over the other is mainly based on results from retrospective analyses of randomized clinical trials and registries. Indeed, a subanalysis of the EXCEL trial comparing PCI with cobalt-chromium fluoropolymer-based everolimus eluting-stents implantation with CABG showed no significant differences between the 2 in terms of death, stroke, and MI in patients with CKD and left main disease.[46] A recent meta-analysis comparing the 2 approaches in diabetic patients with CKD and stable ischemic heart disease showed that CABG on top of optimal medical therapy results in significant reduction in repeat revascularization rate (HR, 0.25; 95%, CI 0.15–0.41; P = .0001), but not in major adverse cardiovascular or cerebrovascular events.[47] Patients on dialysis tend to have better short-term outcomes with PCI but worse long-term outcomes in terms of death, MI, and repeat revascularization.[48] The incidence of acute kidney injury is higher with CABG as compared with PCI, although both interventions are associated with a higher risk of acute kidney injury as compared with patients with normal kidney function.[49]

Contrast-associated nephropathy

Contrast-associated acute kidney injury is one of the most common complications of PCI. It also constitutes a major barrier that prevents patients with impaired kidney function from undergoing invasive revascularization. The incidence of contrast-associated nephropathy in current clinical practice is likely overestimated, especially with the availability of newer less toxic contrast agents (Table 1) and standardized pre- and posthydration techniques. The optimal approach to estimate and minimize the risk of contrast associated acute kidney injury following PCI is discussed elsewhere in this monograph.

Vascular access site in percutaneous coronary interventions

Vascular access site during PCI is another controversial issue surrounding revascularization

Table 1 Contrast agents currently used in PCI				
	Ioxaglate Meglumine and Ioxaglate Sodium (589)	Iopamidol (408, 510, 612, 755)	Iodixanol (550, 652)	Diatrizoate Meglumine and Diatrizoate Sodium
Molecular structure	Ionic dimer	Nonionic monomer	Nonionic dimer	Ionic monomer
Osmolality (mOsm/kg H_2O)	Low 600	Low 413–796	Iso 290	High 1551
Iodine Concentration (mg/mL)	320	200–370	270–320	370
Viscosity (mPa.sec at 37°C)	7.5	2.0–9.4	6.3–11.8	10.5

in patients with CKD. Although a transradial approach is associated with a lower bleeding risk, the transfemoral access site is often preferred, especially in patients with advanced stage kidney disease when the radial artery is needed to make an arteriovenous fistula for dialysis. As for CABG, the Radial Artery Database International Alliance (RADIAL) project showed that the use of radial artery grafts instead of the saphenous vein was associated with a lesser incidence of adverse cardiac events and better graft patency at 5 years of follow-up in patients with preserved renal function, but not in those with CKD. Indeed, a subgroup analysis of patients with renal insufficiency revealed inconclusive results and thus the choice of graft site is made based on each patient's preference.[50]

Dual antiplatelet therapy

Patients with renal impairment who have undergone PCI with stent implantation are at increased risk of postprocedural bleeding and ischemic complications as compared with the general population. Nonetheless, the optimal dual antiplatelet therapy duration in these patients is not well-established, especially among those with advanced disease who are prone to excessive bleeding risks and unclear benefits from an extended duration of dual antiplatelet therapy.[51,52]

ATRIAL FIBRILLATION AND RENAL IMPAIRMENT

Patients with advanced CKD are highly susceptible to various arrhythmias, including atrial flutter, atrial fibrillation (AF), and supraventricular and ventricular arrhythmia.[53] AF is the most prevalent sustained arrhythmia worldwide and could be due to valvular or nonvalvular etiologies, as was shown in the Framingham Heart Study.[54] Indeed, AF is present in around 20%

of patients with CKD and 33% of dialysis-dependent patients with CKD.[55,56] The high prevalence of AF in these patients can be explained by various mechanisms. Early clinical studies showed that plasma catecholamine level is elevated in patients with chronic renal failure leading to a constant activation of the renin–angiotensin–aldosterone system.[57,58] As a result, the circulating angiotensin II level increases, leading to changes in tissue composition, atrial myocytes apoptosis, and subsequent tissue fibrosis.[59] Other potential etiologies include structural changes to the heart, myocardial fibrosis, and ongoing inflammation.[60,61] The end result is the same and includes increased a risk of stroke, progression to end-stage renal disease, and death.[62,63] Stroke is one of the most common complications of AF and results in increased morbidity and mortality.[64] Nonetheless, several stroke prediction risk scores exist and guide prophylactic therapy in these patients. The CHA_2DS_2-VASc (congestive heart failure, hypertension, age 75 years or older, diabetes mellitus, prior stroke, transient ischemic attack, or thromboembolism, vascular disease, age 65 to 74 years, and female sex) has been widely used over the past years for risk stratification and stroke prediction; patients with CKD with a score of 2 or greater benefit from oral anticoagulation.[65]

Impact of Chronic Kidney Disease on the Management of Atrial Fibrillation

Oral anticoagulants (OAC) used in patients with renal impairment are not different from the ones used in the general population (Table 2). OACs are mainly divided into 2 categories: vitamin K antagonists (VKA) and direct OACs. Each has its own pharmacodynamic and pharmacokinetic properties that require special dose adjustments in the presence of kidney dysfunction.

Table 2
Pharmacokinetics of oral anticoagulants used in atrial fibrillation

	Warfarin	Dabigatran	Rivaroxaban	Edoxaban	Apixaban
Mechanism of action	Inhibits production of vitamin K–dependent clotting factors (II, VII, IX, and X)	Inhibits thrombin	Inhibits factor Xa	Inhibits factor Xa	Inhibits factor Xa
Bioavailability	100%	3%–7%	66% without food 80%–100% with food	62%	50% (prolonged absorption)
Time to maximum concentration (hours)	4 (peak anticoagulant effect at 72–96)	1–2	2–4	1–2	3–4
Clearance of absorbed dose (nonrenal/renal)	–	20%/80%	65%/35%	50%/50%	73%/27%
Liver metabolism	Hepatic metabolism	No	Yes (18% hepatic elimination)	Minimal (<4%)	Yes (moderate contribution to elimination, 25%)
Elimination half-life	40 hours	12–17 hours	5–9 hours in young; 11–13 hours in elderly	10–14 hours	12 hours
Reversal	Vitamin K + PCC (or FFP)	Idarucizumab (or PCC)	Andexanet alfa (or PCC)	Andexanet alfa (or PCC)	Andexanet alfa (or PCC)

Abbreviations: FFP, fresh frozen plasma; PCC, prothrombin complex concentrate.

The main mechanism of action of VKAs is inhibition of vitamin K epoxide reductase enzyme that catalyzes the synthesis of coagulation factors in the liver. VKAs have a narrow therapeutic window, exhibit unpredictable dose–response, and interact with the metabolism and elimination of various drugs and foods. Hence, the use of these agents, especially in patients with impaired kidney function, is challenging and requires close monitoring of the prothrombin time. Warfarin is the most commonly used VKA and its efficacy in the prevention of strokes and other systemic embolic events has been well-established in patients with early-stage renal dysfunction.[66] However, warfarin use in late to end-stage kidney disease is not supported by robust evidence and is widely debated in the literature. Indeed, patients with advanced disease have most of the time an international normalized ratio outside the target prophylactic range and thus are constantly at increased risk of stroke and bleeding as compared with patients with milder disease.[67,68]

In contrast, non-vitamin K OACs (NOAC) such as factor Xa inhibitors (rivaroxaban, apixaban, and edoxaban) or thrombin inhibitors (dabigatran) have been shown in several randomized clinical trials to be superior to warfarin in patients with mild to moderate CKD; however, this improvement comes at the expense of increased gastrointestinal bleeding.[69] A recently published systematic review and meta-analysis of 15 studies including 78,053 patients with CKD and treated with OACs for AF showed that NOACs have better safety and efficacy profile for cardiovascular outcomes as compared with warfarin.[70] In adjusted analyses, NOACs use decreased the risk of intracranial hemorrhage (adjusted HR, 0.39; 95% CI, 0.30–0.50) and cerebral or systemic embolism (adjusted HR, 0.75; 95% CI, 0.65–0.88). Moreover, among all NOACs tested, factor Xa inhibitors consistently decreased mortality (relative risk [RR], 0.84; 95% CI, 0.70–1.00), stroke (RR, 0.84; 95% CI, 0.73–0.96), and major bleeding (RR, 0.76; 95% CI, 0.64–0.91).[70] Hence, current clinical guidelines recommend NOACs over VKA in mild-to-moderate disease, yet, the evidence supporting this approach in advanced CKD is weak (Figs. 2).[71,72] Recently, Kuno and colleagues examined the safety and efficacy of OACs in patients with AF and on long-term dialysis in a meta-analysis of 16 studies including a total of 71,877 patients.[73] The authors concluded that OACs' use does not reduce the risk of thromboembolism in patients with AF and advanced kidney disease (apixaban 5 mg, HR= 0.59; 95% CI: 0.30-1.17; apixaban 2.5 mg, HR= 1.00; 95% CI: 0.52-1.93; warfarin, HR= 0.91; 95% CI: 0.72-1.16). Moreover, warfarin was associated with a significantly higher risk of bleeding compared to apixaban or no anticoagulation (vs. apixaban 5 mg, HR= 1.41; 95% CI: 1.07-1.88; vs. apixaban 2.5 mg, HR= 1.40; 95% CI: 1.07-1.82; vs. no anticoagulant, HR= 1.31; 95% CI: 1.15-1.50).[73]

HEART FAILURE AND RENAL IMPAIRMENT

Renal and cardiac functions are tightly interlinked through various humoral, neural, and metabolomic pathways.[74] Renal disease is one of the strongest risk factors for the development of heart failure. Indeed, left ventricular failure is directly affected by 3 fundamental mechanisms, including volume overload, pressure overload, and cardiomyopathy.[4] As kidney function worsens, these 3 parameters become more difficult to control. There are 2 subtypes of heart failure: heart failure with preserved ejection fraction (HFpEF) and heart failure with reduced ejection fraction (HFrEF). HFpEF is highly prevalent in patients with renal disease owing to common underlying comorbidities (ie, obesity, diabetes mellitus, hypertension, dyslipidemia) that increase systemic inflammation and lead to coronary microvascular dysfunction.[75] Nonetheless, no randomized trial showed significant benefits of any therapeutic intervention for HFpEF in patients with renal impairment. In contrast, treatment for HFrEF (ie, β-blockers, angiotensin-converting enzyme inhibitors, angiotensin receptor blockers) in the general population as well as in patients with CKD is supported by strong evidence generated from large, randomized studies. Both subtypes of heart failure are characterized by chronic increases in neurohormonal activity and thus all the therapies target the renin–angiotensin–aldosterone system and other neurohormonal pathways.

Medical Management of Congestive Heart Failure in Patients with Chronic Kidney Disease
Mineralocorticoid antagonists
The mainstay therapeutic agents in heart failure therapy are mineralocorticoid antagonists such as spironolactone and eplerenone (steroidal mineralocorticoid antagonists). In patients with HFrEF with or without kidney disease, spironolactone use decreases all-cause mortality and

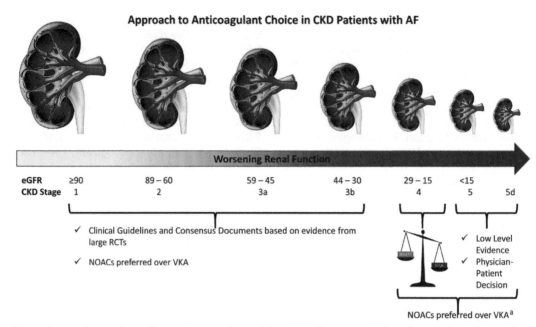

Fig. 2. Approach to anticoagulant choice in patients with atrial fibrillation and kidney disease. [a]Based on evidence from registries. If the risks outweigh the benefits, consider nonpharmacologic therapy (ie, left atrial appendage closure or no therapy). RCT, randomized clinical trial.

hospitalization for heart failure decompensation in the Randomized Aldactone Evaluation Study (RALES).[76] In contrast, the Spironolactone for Heart Failure With Preserved Ejection Fraction (TOPCAT) trial showed that spironolactone is not superior to placebo in improving cardiovascular outcomes in patients with HFpEF.[77] Interestingly, a substudy of the TOPCAT trial showed that, as compared with placebo, spironolactone reduces the risk of cardiovascular outcomes across all estimated GFRs (eGFR), yet, with an increased rate of adverse events (mainly hyperkalemia and worsening kidney function) seen at a low eGFR.[78] Hence, treatment of patients with a low eGFR might be considered if close laboratory monitoring of electrolytes is possible.

Over the past decade, there has been increased interest in the use of nonsteroidal mineralocorticoid antagonists, such as finerenone, owing to a high selectivity for mineralocorticoid receptor and low affinity for androgen and progesterone receptors. Consequently, the side effects associated with spironolactone (ie, gynecomastia, amenorrhea, impotence) could be avoided with finerenone use.[79] The Miner Alocorticoid Receptor antagonist Tolerability Study-Heart Failure (ARTS-HF) study randomized 1066 patients with HFrEF and CKD to either finerenone or eplerenone (a steroidal antimineralocorticoid of the spironolactone group) for

90 days.[80] The level of pro-brain natriuretic peptide, a cardiac hemodynamic stress biomarker, decreased by at least 30% in the experimental arm.[80] Moreover, patients placed on finerenone had a lesser incidence of acute kidney injury as well as hyperkalemia compared with patients who received eplerenone. Indeed, finerenone is a novel drug that holds promise in patients with heart failure with some form of renal impairment.

Neprilysin inhibitors
Another novel class of drugs for heart failure is the combination of an angiotensin receptor blocker, valsartan, and a neprilysin inhibitor, sacubitril, to form valsartan/sacubitril (angiotensin receptor-neprilysin inhibitor [ARNI]). The Prospective Comparison of ARNI with ACEi to Determine Impact on Global Mortality and Morbidity in Heart Failure (PARADIGM-HF, NCT01035255) trial randomized 8442 patients with HFrEF to either sacubitril/valsartan or enalapril.[81] The trial was prematurely terminated owing to overwhelming evidence of sacubitril/valsartan benefits in reduction of cardiovascular death and rehospitalization for heart failure (20% reduction; 95% CI, 13–27) at a median follow-up of 27 months.[81] The benefits of ARNI were observed similarly in patients with and without CKD. After this landmark trial, the European Society of Cardiology 2016 guidelines for

the management of heart failure included valsartan/sacubitril as an alternative for angiotensin converting enzyme inhibitors and angiotensin receptor blockers in patients with a left ventricular ejection fraction of less than 35% and who remain symptomatic despite receiving optimal medical therapy.[82] In contrast, the Prospective Comparison of ARNI With ARB Global Outcomes in HF With Preserved Ejection Fraction (PARAGON-HF, NCT01920711) randomized trial showed that the same approach in patients with HFpEF (left ventricular ejection fraction of ≥45%) did not decrease the incidence of cardiovascular death and rehospitalization for heart failure exacerbation compared with patients treated with valsartan.[83] To note, around 49% of patients enrolled in this trial had an eGFR of less than 60 mL/min/1.73 m^2; from these patients, the experimental group (valsartan/sacubitril) had better outcomes than the control group (valsartan alone) as was shown in a prespecified subgroup analysis (HR, 0.79; 95% CI, 0.66–0.95).[83]

Sodium-glucose co-transporter 2 inhibitors for heart failure

Sodium-glucose co-transporter 2 (SGLT-2) inhibitors are novel glycemic control agents approved for use in type 2 diabetes mellitus. These drugs lower blood sugar level by blocking glucose reabsorption in proximal tubules and thus promote its urinary excretion. In addition, SGLT-2 inhibitors block sodium reabsorption via the same co-transporter in proximal tubules resulting in osmotic diuresis without affecting plasma osmolarity. Owing to this underlying pharmacologic mechanism, SGLT-2 inhibitors use was associated with a significant decrease in cardiovascular adverse events especially in patients with heart failure (**Fig. 3**).[84,85] The EMPA-REG trial (NCT01131676) randomized 7020 diabetic patients with established cardiovascular disease and an eGFR of 30 mL/min/1.73 m^2 or greater to either empagliflozin or placebo once daily. A 34% decrease in cardiovascular death and hospitalization for heart failure was seen in patients on empagliflozin as compared with the placebo group.[86] After this trial, the Canagliflozin Cardiovascular Assessment Study (CANVAS, NCT01032629) enrolled a total of 10,142 diabetic patients at high cardiovascular risk who were then randomized to either canagliflozin or placebo.[87] The primary outcome of interest—a composite of cardiovascular death, nonfatal MI, and nonfatal stroke—occurred in 26.9

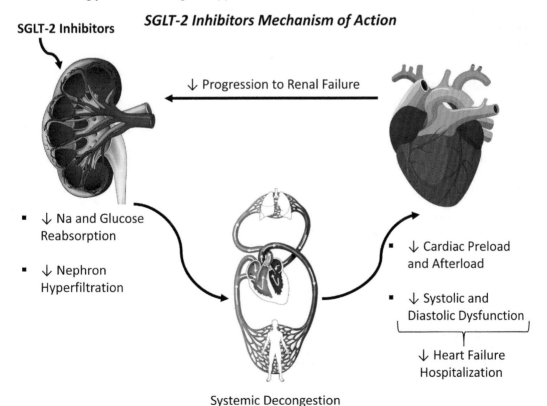

SGLT-2 Inhibitors Mechanism of Action

SGLT-2 Inhibitors

↓ Progression to Renal Failure

- ↓ Na and Glucose Reabsorption
- ↓ Nephron Hyperfiltration

- ↓ Cardiac Preload and Afterload
- ↓ Systolic and Diastolic Dysfunction

↓ Heart Failure Hospitalization

Systemic Decongestion

Fig. 3. Mechanism of action of SGLT-2 inhibitors in heart failure.

(canagliflozin) versus 31.5 (placebo) participants per 1000 patient-years (HR, 0.86; 95% CI, 0.75–0.97; P<.001 for noninferiority; P = .02 for superiority).[87] Furthermore, the study revealed a potential canagliflozin's benefit in slowing down the progression of albuminuria (HR, 0.73; 95% CI, 0.67–0.79) as well as a decrease in the composite outcome of death from renal etiologies, sustained reduction in eGFR, and need for renal replacement therapy (HR, 0.60; 95% CI, 0.47–0.77).[87] However, the results of EMPA-REG and CANVAS trials cannot be generalized to patients with advanced stage renal disease because both studies included patients with a relatively high eGFR (means of 83.1 and 76.5 mL/min/1.73 m^2, respectively) and excluded those with an eGFR of less than 30 mL/min/1.73 m^2.

In a subanalysis of DECLARE-TIMI 58 (NCT01730534) randomized trial, the use of dapagliflozin was shown to prevent progression to renal failure in diabetic patients with or without established atherosclerotic cardiovascular disease.[88] In addition, a prespecified subanalysis from the landmark DAPA-HF (NCT03036124) randomized study showed that dapagliflozin reduces cardiovascular death and hospitalization for heart failure in patients with HFrEF regardless of their kidney function status.[89] Finally, the CREDENCE trial (NCT02065791) showed that, in diabetic patients with established kidney disease, the use of canagliflozin decreases the risk of kidney failure and various cardiovascular events as compared with placebo.[90] Upcoming randomized trials include EMPA-KIDNEY (NCT03594110) study testing the effect of empagliflozin on renal and cardiovascular outcomes in patients with CKD and the DELIVER (NCT03619213) study evaluating the efficacy and safety of dapagliflozin in patients with HFpEF.

FUTURE DIRECTIONS

Owing to an increased incidence of renal function impairment in cardiac patients, management of various cardiovascular diseases should be made through joint decision making between cardiologists and nephrologists. CAD is one of the most common pathologies among patients with kidney disease, yet the evidence supporting the different management strategies is not as strong as the one used for patients with preserved renal function. Randomized clinical trials dedicated for patients with CKD are needed to determine the optimal medical therapy, revascularization modality, and antithrombotic regimen. Newer strategies for the prevention of contrast-induced nephropathy, whether through discovery of less toxic contrast agents or improvement of preconditioning techniques, should also be a main focus of future research.

Similarly, cardiologists do not possess strong evidence that guides anticoagulant choice in patients with AF and decreased kidney function. Hence, their decision follows an individualized approach that takes into consideration patient preferences rather than clinical guidelines. Moreover, risk scores that predict the risk of ischemic and bleeding events based on real-world clinical data from patients with renal impairment are needed.

Finally, the coexistence of heart failure and kidney disease is common among cardiac patients and is often associated with unfavorable clinical outcomes. The underlying heart failure pathophysiology is slightly different from the general population and thus the conventional heart failure therapy might not work similarly in these patients. Novel therapeutic agents, such as SGLT-2 inhibitors and ARNIs, seem to be promising with the increased amount of evidence showing their efficacy in slowing down the deterioration of kidney function. Nonetheless, randomized trials strictly enrolling patients with renal disease are needed to establish the optimal heart failure medical therapy in this population.

REFERENCES

1. Bakris GL, Williams M, Dworkin L, et al. Preserving renal function in adults with hypertension and diabetes: a consensus approach. National Kidney Foundation Hypertension and Diabetes Executive Committees Working Group. Am J Kidney Dis 2000;36:646–61.
2. Geisberg C, Butler J. Addressing the challenges of cardiorenal syndrome. Cleve Clin J Med 2006;73:485.
3. Bright R. Cases and observations illustrative of renal disease accompanied with the secretion of albuminous urine 1836;10:338–40.
4. McCullough PA, Kellum JA, Haase M, et al. Pathophysiology of the cardiorenal syndromes: executive summary from the eleventh consensus conference of the Acute Dialysis Quality Initiative (ADQI). Contrib Nephrol 2013;182:82–98.
5. Ronco C, Haapio M, House AA, et al. Cardiorenal syndrome. J Am Coll Cardiol 2008;52:1527–39.
6. Charrois TL, Zolezzi M, Koshman SL, et al. A systematic review of the evidence for pharmacist care of patients with dyslipidemia. Pharmacotherapy 2012;32:222–33.
7. Briasoulis A, Bakris GL. Chronic kidney disease as a coronary artery disease risk equivalent. Curr Cardiol Rep 2013;15:340.

8. Chonchol M, Whittle J, Desbien A, et al. Chronic kidney disease is associated with angiographic coronary artery disease. Am J Nephrol 2008;28:354–60.

9. Olechnowicz-Tietz S, Gluba A, Paradowska A, et al. The risk of atherosclerosis in patients with chronic kidney disease 2013;45:1605–12.

10. Horowitz B, Miskulin D, Zager P. Epidemiology of hypertension in CKD 2015;22:88–95.

11. Muntner P, Anderson A, Charleston J, et al. Hypertension awareness, treatment, and control in adults with CKD: results from the Chronic Renal Insufficiency Cohort (CRIC) Study. Am J Kidney Dis 2010;55:441–51.

12. Targher G, Chonchol M, Bertolini L, et al. Increased risk of CKD among type 2 diabetics with nonalcoholic fatty liver disease. J Am Soc Nephrol 2008; 19:1564–70.

13. Collins AJ, Vassalotti JA, Wang C, et al. Who should be targeted for CKD screening? Impact of diabetes, hypertension, and cardiovascular disease. Am J Kidney Dis 2009;53:S71–7.

14. Manjunath G, Tighiouart H, Ibrahim H, et al. Level of kidney function as a risk factor for atherosclerotic cardiovascular outcomes in the community. J Am Coll Cardiol 2003;41:47–55.

15. McCullough PA, Li S, Jurkovitz CT, et al. Chronic kidney disease, prevalence of premature cardiovascular disease, and relationship to short-term mortality. Am Heart J 2008;156:277–83.

16. London GM, Guérin AP, Marchais SJ, et al. Arterial media calcification in end-stage renal disease: impact on all-cause and cardiovascular mortality. Nephrol Dial Transplant 2003;18:1731–40.

17. Schwarz U, Buzello M, Ritz E, et al. Morphology of coronary atherosclerotic lesions in patients with end-stage renal failure. Nephrol Dial Transplant 2000;15:218–23.

18. Nakamura S, Ishibashi-Ueda H, Niizuma S, et al. Coronary calcification in patients with chronic kidney disease and coronary artery disease. Clin J Am Soc Nephrol 2009;4:1892–900.

19. Nakano T, Ninomiya T, Sumiyoshi S, et al. Association of kidney function with coronary atherosclerosis and calcification in autopsy samples from Japanese elders: the Hisayama study. Am J Kidney Dis 2010;55:21–30.

20. Campean V, Neureiter D, Varga I, et al. Atherosclerosis and vascular calcification in chronic renal failure. Kidney Blood Press Res 2005;28:280–9.

21. Apostolov EO, Ray D, Savenka AV, et al. Chronic uremia stimulates LDL carbamylation and atherosclerosis. J Am Soc Nephrol 2010;21:1852–7.

22. Sedlis SP, Jurkovitz CT, Hartigan PM, et al. Optimal medical therapy with or without percutaneous coronary intervention for patients with stable coronary artery disease and chronic kidney disease. Am J Cardiol 2009;104:1647–53.

23. Baber U, Mehran R, Kirtane AJ, et al. Prevalence and impact of high platelet reactivity in chronic kidney disease: results from the Assessment of Dual Antiplatelet Therapy with Drug-Eluting Stents registry. Circ Cardiovasc Interv 2015;8:e001683.

24. Sosnov J, Lessard D, Goldberg RJ, et al. Differential symptoms of acute myocardial infarction in patients with kidney disease: a community-wide perspective. Am J Kidney Dis 2006;47:378–84.

25. Herzog CA, Littrell K, Arko C, et al. Clinical characteristics of dialysis patients with acute myocardial infarction in the United States: a collaborative project of the United States Renal Data System and the National Registry of Myocardial Infarction. Circulation 2007;116:1465–72.

26. Burton JO, Jefferies HJ, Selby NM, et al. Hemodialysis-induced repetitive myocardial injury results in global and segmental reduction in systolic cardiac function. Clin J Am Soc Nephrol 2009;4:1925–31.

27. Stefánsson BV, Brunelli SM, Cabrera C, et al. Intradialytic hypotension and risk of cardiovascular disease. Clin J Am Soc Nephrol 2014;9:2124–32.

28. Dobre M, Brateanu A, Rashidi A, et al. Electrocardiogram abnormalities and cardiovascular mortality in elderly patients with CKD. Clin J Am Soc Nephrol 2012;7:949–56.

29. Montague BT, Ouellette JR, Buller GK. Retrospective review of the frequency of ECG changes in hyperkalemia. Clin J Am Soc Nephrol 2008;3:324–30.

30. Wang LW, Fahim MA, Hayen A, et al. Cardiac testing for coronary artery disease in potential kidney transplant recipients. Cochrane Database Syst Rev 2011;(12):CD008691.

31. Wang LW, Fahim MA, Hayen A, et al. Cardiac testing for coronary artery disease in potential kidney transplant recipients: a systematic review of test accuracy studies. Am J Kidney Dis 2011;57:476–87.

32. Patel RK, Mark PB, Johnston N, et al. Prognostic value of cardiovascular screening in potential renal transplant recipients: a single-center prospective observational study. Am J Transplant 2008;8:1673–83.

33. Konstantinidis I, Nadkarni GN, Yacoub R, et al. Representation of patients with kidney disease in trials of cardiovascular interventions: an updated systematic review. JAMA Intern Med 2016;176:121–4.

34. Ridker PM, MacFadyen J, Cressman M, et al. Efficacy of rosuvastatin among men and women with moderate chronic kidney disease and elevated high-sensitivity C-reactive protein: a secondary analysis from the JUPITER (Justification for the Use of Statins in Prevention-an Intervention Trial Evaluating Rosuvastatin) trial. J Am Coll Cardiol 2010;55:1266–73.

35. Fellström BC, Jardine AG, Schmieder RE, et al. Rosuvastatin and cardiovascular events in patients undergoing hemodialysis. N Engl J Med 2009; 360:1395–407.

36. Grundy SM, Stone NJ, Bailey AL, et al. 2018 AHA/ACC/AACVPR/AAPA/ABC/ACPM/ADA/AGS/APhA/ASPC/NLA/PCNA guideline on the management of blood cholesterol: a report of the American College of Cardiology/American Heart Association Task Force on clinical practice guidelines. J Am Coll Cardiol 2019;73:e285–350.

37. Charytan DM, Sabatine MS, Pedersen TR, et al. Efficacy and safety of evolocumab in chronic kidney disease in the FOURIER trial. J Am Coll Cardiol 2019;73:2961–70.

38. Fox CS, Muntner P, Chen AY, et al. Use of evidence-based therapies in short-term outcomes of ST-segment elevation myocardial infarction and non-ST-segment elevation myocardial infarction in patients with chronic kidney disease: a report from the National Cardiovascular Data Acute Coronary Treatment and Intervention Outcomes Network registry. Circulation 2010;121: 357–65.

39. Charytan DM, Wallentin L, Lagerqvist B, et al. Early angiography in patients with chronic kidney disease: a collaborative systematic review. Clin J Am Soc Nephrol 2009;4:1032–43.

40. Bangalore S. International Study of Comparative Health Effectiveness With Medical and Invasive Approaches–Chronic Kidney Disease - ISCHEMIA-CKD. American Heart Association Annual Scientific Sessions (AHA 2019). Philadelphia, PA, 2019.

41. Volodarskiy A, Kumar S, Amin S, et al. Optimal treatment strategies in patients with chronic kidney disease and coronary artery disease. Am J Med 2016;129:1288–98.

42. Hemmelgarn BR, Southern D, Culleton BF, et al. Survival after coronary revascularization among patients with kidney disease. Circulation 2004;110: 1890–5.

43. Reddan DN, Szczech LA, Tuttle RH, et al. Chronic kidney disease, mortality, and treatment strategies among patients with clinically significant coronary artery disease. J Am Soc Nephrol 2003;14:2373–80.

44. Szummer K, Lundman P, Jacobson SH, et al. Influence of renal function on the effects of early revascularization in non-ST-elevation myocardial infarction: data from the Swedish Web-System for Enhancement and Development of Evidence-Based Care in Heart Disease Evaluated According to Recommended Therapies (SWEDEHEART). Circulation 2009;120:851–8.

45. Huang HD, Alam M, Hamzeh I, et al. Patients with severe chronic kidney disease benefit from early revascularization after acute coronary syndrome. Int J Cardiol 2013;168:3741–6.

46. Giustino G, Mehran R, Serruys PW, et al. Left main revascularization with PCI or CABG in patients with chronic kidney disease: EXCEL trial. J Am Coll Cardiol 2018;72:754–65.

47. Farkouh ME, Sidhu MS, Brooks MM, et al. Impact of chronic kidney disease on outcomes of myocardial revascularization in patients with diabetes. J Am Coll Cardiol 2019;73:400–11.

48. Marui A, Kimura T, Nishiwaki N, et al. Percutaneous coronary intervention versus coronary artery bypass grafting in patients with end-stage renal disease requiring dialysis (5-year outcomes of the CREDO-Kyoto PCI/CABG Registry Cohort-2). Am J Cardiol 2014;114:555–61.

49. Chang TI, Leong TK, Boothroyd DB, et al. Acute kidney injury after CABG versus PCI: an observational study using 2 cohorts. J Am Coll Cardiol 2014;64:985–94.

50. Gaudino M, Benedetto U, Fremes S, et al. Radial-artery or saphenous-vein grafts in coronary-artery bypass surgery. N Engl J Med 2018;378:2069–77.

51. Chen Y-T, Chen H-T, Hsu C-Y, et al. Dual antiplatelet therapy and clinical outcomes after coronary drug-eluting stent implantation in patients on hemodialysis. Clin J Am Soc Nephrol 2017; 12:262–71.

52. Palmer SC, Di Micco L, Razavian M, et al. Effects of antiplatelet therapy on mortality and cardiovascular and bleeding outcomes in persons with chronic kidney disease: a systematic review and meta-analysis. Ann Intern Med 2012;156:445–59.

53. Roberts PR, Green D. Arrhythmias in chronic kidney disease. Heart 2011;97:766–73.

54. Benjamin EJ, Levy D, Vaziri SM, et al. Independent risk factors for atrial fibrillation in a population-based cohort. The Framingham Heart Study. JAMA 1994;271:840–4.

55. Wetmore JB, Mahnken JD, Rigler SK, et al. The prevalence of and factors associated with chronic atrial fibrillation in Medicare/Medicaid-eligible dialysis patients. Kidney Int 2012;81:469–76.

56. Ananthapanyasut W, Napan S, Rudolph EH, et al. Prevalence of atrial fibrillation and its predictors in nondialysis patients with chronic kidney disease. Clin J Am Soc Nephrol 2010;5:173–81.

57. Beretta-Piccoli C, Weidmann P, Schiffl H, et al. Enhanced cardiovascular pressor reactivity to norepinephrine in mild renal parenchymal disease. Kidney Int 1982;22:297–303.

58. Ishii M, Ikeda T, Takagi M, et al. Elevated plasma catecholamines in hypertensives with primary glomerular diseases. Hypertension 1983;5:545–51.

59. Burstein B, Nattel S. Atrial fibrosis: mechanisms and clinical relevance in atrial fibrillation. J Am Coll Cardiol 2008;51:802–9.

60. Hung M-J, Yang N-I, Wu IW, et al. Echocardiographic assessment of structural and functional

cardiac remodeling in patients with predialysis chronic kidney disease. Echocardiography 2010; 27:621–9.

61. Nattel S. Molecular and cellular mechanisms of atrial fibrosis in atrial fibrillation. JACC Clin Electrophysiol 2017;3:425–35.

62. Bansal N, Fan D, Hsu CY, et al. Incident atrial fibrillation and risk of end-stage renal disease in adults with chronic kidney disease. Circulation 2013; 127(5):569–74.

63. Bansal N, Fan D, Hsu CY, et al. Incident atrial fibrillation and risk of death in adults with chronic kidney disease. J Am Heart Assoc 2014;3(5):e001303.

64. Bansal N, Xie D, Sha D, et al. Cardiovascular events after new-onset atrial fibrillation in adults with CKD: results from the chronic renal insufficiency cohort (CRIC) study. J Am Soc Nephrol 2018;29(12):2859–69.

65. Melgaard L, Gorst-Rasmussen A, Lane DA, et al. Assessment of the CHA2DS2-VASc score in predicting ischemic stroke, thromboembolism, and death in patients with heart failure with and without atrial fibrillation. JAMA 2015;314(10):1030–8.

66. Hart RG, Pearce LA, Asinger RW, et al. Warfarin in atrial fibrillation patients with moderate chronic kidney disease. Clin J Am Soc Nephrol 2011;6(11): 2599–604.

67. Yang F, Hellyer JA, Than C, et al. Warfarin utilisation and anticoagulation control in patients with atrial fibrillation and chronic kidney disease. Heart 2017;103(11):818–26.

68. Limdi NA, Beasley TM, Baird MF, et al. Kidney function influences warfarin responsiveness and hemorrhagic complications. J Am Soc Nephrol 2009;20(4): 912–21.

69. Ruff CT, Giugliano RP, Braunwald E, et al. Comparison of the efficacy and safety of new oral anticoagulants with warfarin in patients with atrial fibrillation: a meta-analysis of randomised trials. Lancet 2014;383(9921):955–62.

70. Malhotra K, Ishfaq MF, Goyal N, et al. Oral anticoagulation in patients with chronic kidney disease: a systematic review and meta-analysis. Neurology 2019;92(21):e2421–31.

71. Steffel J, Verhamme P, Potpara TS, et al. The 2018 European Heart Rhythm Association Practical Guide on the use of non-vitamin K antagonist oral anticoagulants in patients with atrial fibrillation. Eur Heart J 2018;39(16):1330–93.

72. January CT, Wann LS, Calkins H, et al. 2019 AHA/ACC/HRS Focused Update of the 2014 AHA/ACC/HRS guideline for the management of patients with atrial fibrillation: a report of the American College of Cardiology/American Heart Association Task Force on Clinical Practice Guidelines and the Heart Rhythm Society [published correction appears in J Am Coll Cardiol. 2019 Jul 30;74(4):599]. J Am Coll Cardiol 2019;74(1):104–32.

73. Kuno T, Takagi H, Ando T. Oral anticoagulation for patients with atrial fibrillation on long-term hemodialysis. J Am Coll Cardiol 2020;75:273–85.

74. Ronco C, Cicoira M, McCullough PA. Cardiorenal syndrome type 1: pathophysiological crosstalk leading to combined heart and kidney dysfunction in the setting of acutely decompensated heart failure. J Am Coll Cardiol 2012;60(12):1031–42.

75. Paulus WJ, Tschöpe C. A novel paradigm for heart failure with preserved ejection fraction: comorbidities drive myocardial dysfunction and remodeling through coronary microvascular endothelial inflammation. J Am Coll Cardiol 2013;62(4):263–71.

76. Pitt B, Zannad F, Remme WJ, et al. The effect of spironolactone on morbidity and mortality in patients with severe heart failure. Randomized Aldactone Evaluation Study Investigators. N Engl J Med 1999;341(10):709–17.

77. Pitt B, Pfeffer MA, Assmann SF, et al. Spironolactone for heart failure with preserved ejection fraction. N Engl J Med 2014;370(15):1383–92.

78. Beldhuis IE, Myhre PL, Claggett B, et al. Efficacy and safety of spironolactone in patients with HFpEF and chronic kidney disease. JACC Heart Fail 2019; 7(1):25–32.

79. Braunschweig F, Linde C, Benson L, et al. New York Heart Association functional class, QRS duration, and survival in heart failure with reduced ejection fraction: implications for cardiac resynchronization therapy. Eur J Heart Fail 2017;19(3):366–76.

80. Filippatos G, Anker SD, Böhm M, et al. A randomized controlled study of finerenone vs. eplerenone in patients with worsening chronic heart failure and diabetes mellitus and/or chronic kidney disease. Eur Heart J 2016; 37(27):2105–14.

81. McMurray JJ, Packer M, Desai AS, et al. Angiotensin-neprilysin inhibition versus enalapril in heart failure. N Engl J Med 2014;371(11):993–1004.

82. Ponikowski P, Voors AA, Anker SD, et al. 2016 ESC guidelines for the diagnosis and treatment of acute and chronic heart failure: The Task Force for the diagnosis and treatment of acute and chronic heart failure of the European Society of Cardiology (ESC) Developed with the special contribution of the Heart Failure Association (HFA) of the ESC. Eur Heart J 2016;37(27):2129–200 [Erratum appears in Eur Heart J. 2016 Dec 30].

83. Solomon SD, McMurray JJV, Anand IS, et al. Angiotensin-neprilysin inhibition in heart failure with preserved ejection fraction. N Engl J Med 2019; 381(17):1609–20.

84. Wu JH, Foote C, Blomster J, et al. Effects of sodium-glucose cotransporter-2 inhibitors on cardiovascular events, death, and major safety outcomes in adults with type 2 diabetes: a systematic review and meta-analysis. Lancet Diabetes

Endocrinol 2016;4(5):411–9 [Erratum appears in Lancet Diabetes Endocrinol. 2016 Sep;4(9):e9].

85. Gilbert RE, Krum H. Heart failure in diabetes: effects of anti-hyperglycaemic drug therapy. Lancet 2015;385(9982):2107–17.

86. Zinman B, Wanner C, Lachin JM, et al. Empagliflozin, cardiovascular outcomes, and mortality in type 2 diabetes. N Engl J Med 2015;373(22):2117–28.

87. Neal B, Perkovic V, Mahaffey KW, et al. Canagliflozin and cardiovascular and renal events in type 2 diabetes. N Engl J Med 2017;377(7):644–57.

88. Mosenzon O, Wiviott SD, Cahn A, et al. Effects of dapagliflozin on development and progression of kidney disease in patients with type 2 diabetes: an analysis from the DECLARE-TIMI 58 randomised trial. Lancet Diabetes Endocrinol 2019;7(8):606–17 [Erratum appears in Lancet Diabetes Endocrinol. 2019 Aug;7(8):e20].

89. Solomon et al. 2019 The Dapaglifozin in Heart Failure with Reduced Ejection Fraction trial (DAPA-HF): outcomes in patients with CKD and effects on renal function. Presented at the American Society of Nephrology Kidney Week 2019 (ASN 2019); November 5–10, Washington, DC, Abstract #FR-OR133.

90. Perkovic V, Jardine MJ, Neal B, et al. Canagliflozin and renal outcomes in type 2 diabetes and nephropathy. N Engl J Med 2019;380(24):2295–306.

Contrast Media—Different Types of Contrast Media, Their History, Chemical Properties, and Relative Nephrotoxicity

Sadichhya Lohani, MD*, Michael R. Rudnick, MD

KEYWORDS

- Contrast-induced nephropathy • Contrast media • High osmolar • Low osmolar • Iso-osmolar
- Contrast-induced acute kidney injury

KEY POINTS

- The hypothesis of osmolality as a cause of injection pain led to the discovery of low-osmolar contrast media (LOCM) and iso-osmolar contrast media (IOCM) and discontinuation of earlier high-osmolar contrast media (HOCM).
- The evidence from many clinical studies has failed to support initial claims that IOCM is less nephrotoxic than LOCM.
- The lack of significant difference in CIN with IOCM and LOCM led to the concepts that osmolality is likely not the only cause of CIN and that other chemical properties like viscosity also contribute to the risk.
- In vivo and in vitro model results do not necessarily translate into human toxicity, as shown by results of clinical studies.

INTRODUCTION

Contrast-induced nephropathy (CIN) is defined as acute kidney injury (AKI) caused by the iodinated contrast media (CM) within 48 hours to 72 hours after CM administration. Chronic kidney disease (CKD), with an estimated glomerular filtration rate (GFR) less than 30 mL/min/1.73 m^2 to 45 mL/min/1.73 m^2, and diabetes mellitus (DM) are the most predictive CIN risk factors, regardless of the CM used. The history and evolution of chemical and osmolar characteristics of different CM are important in understanding the pathophysiology and prevention of CIN. Avoidance of high-osmolar CM (HOCM), use of lowest volume of CM, and volume optimization with isotonic fluids are important preventative measures.

HISTORY AND CHEMICAL PROPERTIES OF CONTRAST MEDIA

In 1896, Wilhelm Roentgen invented radiographs.[1,2] Shortly thereafter, Hashek and Lindenthal used calcium and mercury compounds to perform the first angiography in an amputated hand.[3] Initial investigators realized that elements with high atomic numbers would enhance tissue on x-ray images. Bismuth, lead, barium salts, and other elements initially were evaluated as CM but all were abandoned due to toxicity.[1,4–6]

Renal-Electrolyte and Hypertension Division, Penn Presbyterian Medical Center, Perelman School of Medicine, University of Pennsylvania, 51N 39th Market Street, Suite 240, Philadelphia, PA 19104, USA
* Corresponding author.
E-mail address: sadichhya.lohani@pennmedicine.upenn.edu
Twitter: @LohaniSadichhya (S.L.); @MichaelRudnick7 (M.R.R.)

Intervent Cardiol Clin 9 (2020) 279–292
https://doi.org/10.1016/j.iccl.2020.02.008
2211-7458/20/© 2020 Elsevier Inc. All rights reserved.

A solution of sodium iodide was first used by Cameron in 1918.[2,7] In the early 1920s, Osborne and colleagues[8] noted that urine of syphilis patients treated with iodine compounds was radiopaque. Uroselectan and diodrast, iodinated derivatives of iodopyridine (a 5-carbon ring molecule), were the earliest CM used worldwide.[4,9,10] In 1933, Wallingford produced the iodine pyridine derivative, para-aminohippuric acid, incorporating up to 3 iodine atoms per molecule.[4,11,12] Wallingord and Swick next introduced a 6-carbon benzene ring as the iodine carrier leading to the development of acetrizoate (Urokon) in 1951, the first true iodinated benzoic acid derivative.[13] In 1953, diatrizoic acid (Hypaque) as the sodium or meglumine salt was developed, followed by the development of iothalamate and metrizoate (Fig. 1).[1,11,14] These early CM were ionic, containing a sodium or meglumine atom that dissociated in aqueous solution from a benzene ring molecule carrying 3 iodine atoms. Because these ionic CM required 2 osmotically active particles to deliver 3 iodine atoms, this resulted in extremely high osmolality of approximately 2000 mOsm/L; thus, these CM have been termed, HOCM.[15] HOCM remained in use until late 1980s but are used uncommonly today for intravascular imaging due to increased nephrotoxicity, injection pain, and high adverse reactions.[4,16,17] Diatrizoic sodium and meglumine (Gastrografin) are still used as oral CM.[18]

Almén suggested that the high osmolality of the then current CM could be reduced by substituting the ionized carboxyl radical in the benzene ring with a nonionized amide (CONH₂) radical, reducing the osmolality of the CM molecule by 50%.[13,17,19,20] CM developed from this concept are now termed, nonionic low-osmolar CM (LOCM), and, because they have a single nonionic benzene ring, also are classified as a monomer.[13,17,20,21] The first LOCM developed in 1970s was metrizamide (Amipaque) but its use was limited because it precipitated at high sterilization temperatures.[4,13] This problem resolved with subsequent formulations of LOCM. The LOCM iohexol (Omnipaque), iopamidol (Isovue) (Fig. 2A), and ioxaglate (Hexabrix) (Fig. 2B) were Food and Drug Administration (FDA) approved in 1985 followed by the approval of ioversol (Optiray) in 1988 and iopromide (Ultravist) in 2002.[22] Ioxaglate (Hexabrix) is unique in that although it is an ionic CM, it is still able to be grouped with the LOCM because each molecule contains 2 benzene rings (a dimer), with a total of 6 iodine atoms.

In order to reduce osmolality further, a new class of CM was developed by attaching 2 nonionic benzene rings to produce a dimer, each containing 3 atoms of iodine, resulting in each osmotically active molecule having 6 iodine atoms.[23] Due to the reduction in molecules needed to deliver the optimal iodine concentration, the osmolality of this CM was reduced and is iso-osmolar (290 mOsm/kg H₂O) to plasma, termed, iso-osmolar CM (IOCM). This reduction in osmolality, however, comes with the price of increased viscosity.[24] The only IOCM approved by the FDA (approval 1996) is iodixanol (Visipaque) (Fig. 3).[25]

To summarize, CM vary in terms of osmolality, viscosity, and ionic/nonionic properties. The differences in the number of atoms per unit volume between an object and its surroundings creates an object contrast.[1] Iodine content in relation to osmotic particle per molecule is important in attenuation.[13,21,26] The CM ratio is the number of iodine atoms divided by number of particles in a solution—the higher the ratio, the lower the osmolality of the CM.[1,13,21] Table 1 is a summary of the various CM and their properties.

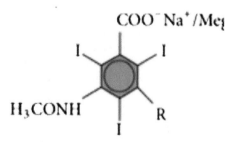

Fig. 1. Structures of HOCM iothalamate and sodium diatrizoate. HOCM have an iodine-to-molecule ratio of 1.5:1. (From Solomon R. Contrast media: are there differences in nephrotoxicity among contrast media? BioMed research international. 2014;2014:934947; with permission.)

EMERGENCE OF LOW-OSMOLAR CONTRAST MEDIA AND IMPACT ON NEPHROTOXICITY

CM was first reported to cause AKI in 1954 when Bartels and colleagues[27] reported a patient who developed anuria after intravenous pyelography. Later, more reports on AKI after CM administration during coronary angiography began to be published and the term, CIN, was defined. The American College of Radiology (ACR) has suggested replacing the term, CIN, with the term, contrast-induced AKI (CI-AKI). The ACR introduced the term, postcontrast AKI (PC-AKI), for AKI after CM exposure in which it is uncertain

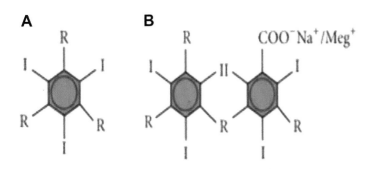

A

B

Fig. 2. Structures of LOCM. (A) Chemical structure of LOCM, nonionic, and monomer (iohexol, ioversol, and iopamidol). LOCM have an iodine-to-molecule ratio of 3:1. (B) Structure of LOCM ionic dimer (ioxaglate). (From Solomon R. Contrast media: are there differences in nephrotoxicity among contrast media? BioMed research international. 2014;2014:934947; with permission.)

if the CM caused the AKI.[28] CIN results in significant morbidity and mortality in hospitalized patients and has been observed to be the third leading cause of hospital-acquired AKI.[29,30] As discussed previously, HOCM were the standard CM until LOCM were introduced in 1980s, with the latter eventually replacing HOCM due to the reduced incidence of adverse events and cost.[17,31]

The primary mechanisms by which CM cause AKI are by causing renal ischemia and by direct tubular epithelial cell toxicity.[32] CM reduce the oxygen tension in the medulla, as a result of increased work of active transport in response to an osmotic diuresis from hyperosmolar agents as well as the release of vasoconstrictive compounds, such as endothelin.[33] In addition, this contrast-induced medullary hypoxic injury is exacerbated by the blockade of vasodilatory compounds, such as nitrous oxide (NO) and prostaglandins.[33] These hypoxic injuries result in reactive oxygen species, which mediate AKI.

Experimental observations suggest that the hyperosmolality and ionic composition of CM play roles in the pathogenesis of CIN.[34–36] Animal studies suggested HOCM were much more

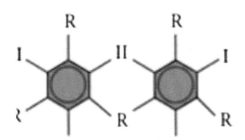

Fig. 3. Chemical structure of IOCM: iodixanol (Visipaque). IOCM have an iodine-to-molecule ratio of 6:1. (From Solomon R. Contrast media: are there differences in nephrotoxicity among contrast media? BioMed research international. 2014;2014:934947; with permission.)

nephrotoxic than LOCM.[37] LOCM cause less reduction in renal blood flow,[38–43] albuminuria,[41,44–46] enzymuria,[46,47] GFR,[37,41,47] and histologic damage.[40,47–49] Based on these experimental observations of reduced nephrotoxicity, the introduction of LOCM into clinical practice was quickly followed by the hope that LOCM would be less nephrotoxic than HOCM. Initial clinical studies on this issue, however, failed to demonstrate a difference in the incidence of nephrotoxicity between HOCM and LOCM.[50–56] These studies were limited, however, by small number of high-risk patients for CIN, that is, patients with preexisting CKD with or without DM. Based on these limitations, it was not possible to assess the relative nephrotoxicity between the LOCM and HOCM groups in these initial studies.[57]

Subsequently, a randomized prospective study comparing the CIN incidence between the LOCM iohexol and the HOCM diatrizoate was performed in a large patient population (1196) undergoing coronary angiography. This study included both low-risk (normal renal function without DM [30.4%] and with DM [26.6%]) and high-risk (CKD without DM [24.9%] and with DM [18.1%]) patients.[57] The iohexol was associated with significantly less nephrotoxicity than the diatrizoate in high-risk azotemic patients.[57] In nonazotemic patients, however, with or without DM, there was no reduction in nephrotoxicity with iohexol compared with diatrizoate—not surprising because patients with normal renal function are not at risk for CIN.[57] A meta-analysis at approximately the same time also concluded that LOCM are less nephrotoxic than HOCM in patients with preexisting CKD.[35] Based on these studies, it was recommended that LOCM be used in patients at high risk for CIN-CKD with or without DM.[49] Shortly after these observations, the costs of LOCM became comparable to HOCM and LOCM became the standard CM used in patients who

Table 1
Summary of contrast media and their chemical properties

Generic Name	Brand Name	Type	Chemical Property	Number of Iodine Atoms per Molecule in Solution	Osmolality, mOsm/kg H_2O	Viscosity, 37° C (cP [mPa·s])	Monomer or Dimer
Iothalamate	Conray-30 Conray-43 Conray	HOCM	Ionic	6	600 1000 1400	4	Monomer
Diatrizoate meglumine/sodium	Gastrografin MD-Gastroview MD-76	HOCM	Ionic	6	1940 2000 1551	10.5	Monomer
Ioxaglate	Hexabrix	LOCM	Ionic	3	~600	7.5	Dimer
Iodipamide	Cholografin	LOCM	Ionic	3	664		Dimer
Iopamidol	Isovue-200 Isovue-250 Isovue-300 Isovue-370	LOCM	Nonionic	3	413 524 616 796	4.7	Monomer
Iopromide	Ultravist-150 Ultravist-240 Ultravist-300 Ultravist-370	LOCM	Nonionic	3	328 483 610 774	4.9	Monomer
Ioversol	Optiray-240 Optiray-300 Optiray-320 Optiray-350	LOCM	Nonionic	3	502 651 702 792	5.5	Monomer
Ioxilan	Oxilan-300 Oxilan-350	LOCM	Nonionic	3	610 721	5.1	Monomer
Iohexol	Omnipaque-140 Omnipaque-180 Omnipaque-240 Omnipaque-300 Omnipaque-350	LOCM	Nonionic	3	322 408 520 672 844	6.3	Monomer
Iodixanol	Visipaque-270 Visipaque-320	IOCM	Nonionic	1.5	290 290	6.3 11.8	Dimer

American College of Radiology Manual on CM, Version 10.3. 2018.
Abbreviations: HOCM, high osmolar Contrast Media; IOCM, iso osmolar contrast Media; LOCM, low osmolar contrast Media.
From ACR Manual on Contrast Media. 11th ed. ACR. ACR Committee on Drugs and Contrast, USA, 2020; with permission.

required intravascular CM due to their lower adverse event profile, regardless of risk of CIN. The incidence of CIN with LOCM is low in the general population (<2%).[58] During coronary angiography, CKD patients, especially if they also have DM, are at increased risk; incidence rates range from 12% to 50%.[51,52,59–65]

ISO-OSMOLAR CONTRAST MEDIA AND CONTRAST-INDUCED NEPHROPATHY— CLINICAL STUDIES

As discussed previously, iodixanol (Visipaque) is the only IOCM available in the United States.[59,66] Based on studies that demonstrated that LOCM were less nephrotoxic than HOCM in high-risk patients, studies were conducted with the hope of demonstrating that IOCM would be less nephrotoxic than LOCM. Table 2 summarizes many of the larger studies of CIN comparing LOCM with IOCM.

Similar to the studies in Table 2, several other studies have failed to demonstrate a reduced CIN risk with IOCM compared with LOCM.[58,67–72] Given the large number of trials that have evaluated CIN risk between LOCM and IOCM, several systematic reviews and meta-analyses comparing the nephrotoxicity of iodixanol to LOCM have been published.[66,73–85] A meta-analysis by Heinrich and colleagues[75] using data pooled from 25 trials (3270 patients) found no difference in the CIN rate between iodixanol and LOCM. When comparing studies using a specific LOCM, CIN risk was greater for iohexol than for iodixanol with intraarterial administration and renal insufficiency (relative risk [RR] 0.38; 95% CI: 0.21-0.68), whereas there was no difference between iodixanol and the other (noniohexol) LOCM (RR 0.95; 95% CI: 0.50-1.78).[75] It is possible that iohexol carries an increased CIN risk compared with noniohexol LOCM, because studies have shown a decreased AKI risk with iodixanol compared with iohexol versus when compared with noniohexol LOCM.[59,76,86–88]

Eng and colleagues[66] reviewed 25 randomized controlled trials (RCTs) for iodixanol with LOCM (5053 patients); 18 studies with intraarterial and 7 with intravenous CM use (Fig. 4). In this meta-analysis, a slight reduction in CIN risk was noted with iodixanol compared with a diverse group of LOCM that just reached statistical significance (pooled RR 0.80; 95% [CI: 0.65-0.99]; P = .045). The point estimate of this reduction, however, did not exceed a minimally important RR difference of 0.25; hence, the lower did not exceed a minimally important

clinical difference. No difference in comparative CIN risk was noted based on route of administration (intra-arterial pooled RR 0.80; 95% [CI: 0.64-1.01]; P = .059]; intravenous 0.84; 95% [CI: 0.42-1.71]; P = .64]).[66] No differences were found in CIN risk among types of LOCM 1 one LOCM was not superior to another in the systematic review and in a small RCT.[66,89–93]

Iodixanol has not been shown be superior to LOCM for cardiovascular events, as demonstrated in a meta-analysis of RCTs comparing iodixanol and LOCM that included cardiac events (cardiac death, coronary artery bypass graft, myocardial infarction, repeat percutaneous coronary intervention [PCI], stroke, thromboembolic event, angina pectoris, arrhythmia, dyspnea, and ventricular extrasystoles).[82] In a more recent metanalysis of 8 prospective RCTs studying iodixanol and LOCM iopromide only (3532 patients), there was no significant difference in the CIN incidence between iodixanol and iopromide (odds ratio [OR] 0.50; 95% CI: 0.19-1.35; P = 0.17).[83] Iodixanol was associated, however, with a statistically significant reduction in cardiovascular adverse events compared with iopromide (OR 0.47; 95% [CI: 0.30-0.73; P = 0.0009]) but only 104 cardiovascular events were recorded from both groups, limiting the clinical implications of this finding.[83]

In a meta-analysis of 12 prospective trials (952 patients) by Han and colleagues[84] only in DM patients, there was no statistically significant reduction of incident CIN associated with iodixanol compared with LOCM iohexol (RR 0.72; 95% [CI: 0.49-1.04; P = .08]). In another recent meta-analysis by Zhao, 15 prospective RCTs, including 2190 DM patients with or without CKD receiving iodixanol or an LOCM, were evaluated. Again, there was no significant difference in CIN between the IOCM and LOCM groups (OR 1.66; 95% [CI: 0.97-2.94; P = .06]). Similar findings were noted when only DM with CKD were included. When CIN was defined only by an increase of serum creatinine (SCr) greater than or equal to 0.5 mg/dL, however, less nephrotoxicity was noted with IOCM compared with LOCM (OR 2.77; 95% [CI: 1.09-7.05; P = .03]). Only 82 total patients, however, developed CIN from both groups making the clinical significance of this observation unclear.[85]

ISO-OSMOLAR CONTRAST MEDIA AND CONTRAST-INDUCED NEPHROPATHY— EXPERIMENTAL STUDIES

A proposed hypothesis for less nephrotoxicity with IOCM is less osmolar diuresis with these

Table 2
Summary of studies on contrast-induced nephropathy incidence between the iso-osmolar contrast media iodixanol versus low-osmolar contrast media

Author, Year	Low-Osmolar Contrast Media	Chronic Kidney Disease (N)	Diabetes Mellitus (%)	Mean Serum Creatinine (mg/dL)	Definition of Contrast-Induced Nephropathy	Indication for Contrast Media	Contrast-Induced Nephropathy Rate (%)	Comments
Chalmers & Jackson,[110] 1999	Iohexol	102	3	IOCM: 3.05 LOCM: 3.34	Scr ↑ >10%	RA, PA	IOCM: 15 LOCM: 31 (P<.005)	Very sensitive definition CIN—loss of specificity
Aspelin et al,[86] 2003	Iohexol	129	100	IOCM: 1.49 LOCM: 1.60	Scr ≥0.5 mg/dL	CA, PA	IOCM: 3 LOCM: 26 (P = .002)	Greatest ↓ CIN with IOCM of all studies—magnitude not duplicated in subsequent studies
McCullough et al,[73] 2006	Iohexol Iopamidol Iopromide Ioxaglate	735	21	CKD IOCM: 1.43 LOCM:1.50	SCr ↑ 0.5 mg/dL	CA, PA	CKD IOCM: 1.4 LOCM: 3.5 (P = .001) CKD and DM: IOCM: 3.5 LOCM: 15.5 (P = .003)	Limitations: inclusion nonpublished data and grouping of multiple LOCM
Solomon et al,[88] 2007	Iopamidol	482	40	IOCM: 1.44 ± 0.41 LOCM: 1.46 ± 0.36	SCr ≥ 0.5 mg/dL	CA	CKD IOCM: 6.7 LOCM: 4.4 (P = .39) CKD and DM: IOCM: 13 LOCM: 5.1 (P = .11)	Major adverse events > for IOCM
	Ioversol	337	52		Scr ↑ ≥0.5 mg/dL		IOCM: 22	

Rudnick et al,[59] 2008				IOCM: 1.99 LOCM: 1.92		CA ± PCI	LOCM: 24 (P = .78)	Premature termination trial due to ↑CIN in NAC patients → underpowered
Laskey et al,[87] 2009	Iopamidol	526	100	IOCM: 1.63 LOCM:1.6	SCr ↑ 0.5 mg/dL	CA	IOCM: 11 LOCM: 10 (P = .7)	No difference in CIN between IOCM and LOCM

Abbreviations: CA, coronary angiography; CKD, chronic kidney disease; CIN, contrast induced nephropathy; DM, diabetes mellitus; IOCM, iso osmolar contrast Media; LOCM, low osmolar contrast Media; N, number of patients; PA, peripheral and aortic angiography; RA, renal angiography; SCr, serum creatinine.

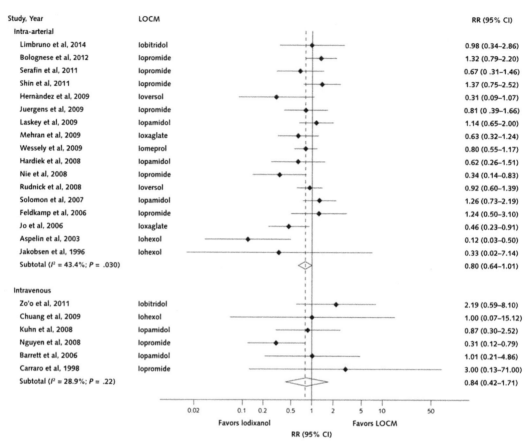

Fig. 4. Graphic summary of meta-analysis of RCTs comparing iodixanol and LOCM with CIN as the primary outcome. The solid vertical line represents the null hypothesis (RR = 1), and the dashed vertical line represents the pooled estimate from the meta-analysis. Studies are shown in reverse chronologic order, grouped by route of administration. CI, confidence interval; LOCM, low osmolar contrast Media; RR, relative risk. (*From* Weisberg LS, Kurnik PB, Kurnik BR. Risk of radiocontrast nephropathy in patients with and without diabetes mellitus. *Kidney international.* 1994;45(1):259-265; with permission.)

agents compared with LOCM. Osmolar diuresis increases distal sodium delivery, which in turn increases oxygen requirement required in the reabsorption of sodium in the thick ascending limb of the loop of Henle producing hypoxia as well as volume depletion along with activation of vasoregulatory hormones. These regulatory mechanisms are significantly impaired in patients with DM and CKD, explaining the increased nephrotoxicity of these subgroups.[32,86,94] Despite these advantages of lower osmolality, animal studies comparing IOCM with LOCM have not for the most part demonstrated a lower rate of renal abnormalities with the IOCM, possibly because of the adverse effects of increased viscosity.[24,34,95,96] Experimental studies in rats suggest that the high viscosity of dimeric CM might be a risk factor by causing red cells sludging in the vasa recta of the renal tubules and other small renal vessels contributing to outer medullary ischemia.[97]

In 1 study, iodixanol significantly decreased outer medullary vasa rectae vasoconstriction along with decreasing NO bioavailability.[98] In another study, iodixanol caused significantly greater increase in urine viscosity than LOCM iopromide and depressed GFR, whereas iopromide did not affect the GFR. Saline attenuated these effects of iodixanol, possibly explaining the protective effects of volume expansion in CIN.[99] Blood oxygenation level–dependent (BOLD) imaging and diffusion-weighted imaging are magnetic resonance imaging techniques to assess renal oxygenation. In a study using BOLD techniques, iodixanol compared with iopromide caused increased hypoxia in the outer medullary area.[100] Other studies using BOLD techniques have demonstrated similar adverse effects on medullary blood flow and oxygen levels with iodixanol.[101–103]

Not all experimental studies, however, demonstrate increased nephrotoxicity of iodixanol compared with LOCM. In a partially nephrectomized animal model, iohexol compared with iodixanol induced a significantly greater reduction in renal function, severe renal tissue damage, intrarenal hypoxia, and apoptotic tubular cells.[104] Cheng and colleagues[105] demonstrated that iohexol induced more severe nephrotoxicity than iodixanol in vivo due to apoptosis, destruction of antioxidative defense, activation of NLRP3 inflammasome, mitochondrial damage, and mitophagy. These results are consistent with clinical observations demonstrating reduced nephrotoxicity of iodixanol compared with iohexol.

Even though experimental studies have been divided, with some literature supporting[73,106] and some not supporting[68,69,107,108] the hypothesis of reduced nephrotoxicity with iodixanol compared with LOCM, overwhelming evidence with many clinical studies and systematic reviews has failed to show that iodixanol is less nephrotoxic than LOCM. Hence, currently the choice of IOCM versus LOCM in practice depends on cost and institution preference.[83] The

Table 3		
Summary of society guidelines about type of contrast media		
Society	**Guideline**	**Comments**
Acute Kidney Injury Work Group, 2012[111]	Recommends using either IOCM or LOCM, rather than HOCM in patients at increased risk of CI-AKI. (1B) Use the lowest possible CM dose in patients at risk for CI-AKI (not graded)	Does not favor IOCM vs LOCM
American College of Cardiology/American Heart Association	PCI focused update 2009: In CKD patients not on chronic dialysis undergoing angiography, either an IOCM (level of evidence A) or a LOCM other than ioxaglate or iohexol is indicated (level of evidence B)[112] 2011: insufficient strength and consistency of relationships between IOCM or LOCM and CIN to enable guideline statement on selection among IOCM and LOCM[113]	2007 guideline on IOCM use in high-risk patients, now deleted Current guidelines recommend focusing on hydration and minimizing contrast volume; does not favor IOCM vs LOCM
European Society of Urogenital Radiology, 2011[114]	No evidence that IOCM are associated with a significantly lower PC-AKI than LOCM. Avoid HOCM.	Recommends using the lowest dose of either LOCM or IOCM
ACR, 2018[28]	LOCM—less nephrotoxic than HOCM in patients with renal insufficiency CIN in LOCM not significantly different in patients with normal renal function Studies failed to establish a clear advantage of iodixanol over LOCM regarding PC-AKI or CIN.	Does not favor IOCM vs LOCM
UpToDate[115]	Use iodixanol or LOCM- iopamidol or ioversol vs iohexol in patients at CIN risk. Avoid HOCM.	

Abbreviations: ACR, American college of radiology; CIN, contrast induced nephropathy; CKD, chronic kidney disease, CM, contrast media; HOCM, high osmolar contrast media; IOCM, iso osmolar contrast media; LOCM, low osmolar contrast media; PC-AKI, post contrast acute kidney injury.

cost of iodixanol in many centers is significantly higher than the cost of LOCM.

SOCIETY GUIDELINES

Based on the cumulative experimental and clinical data comparing the nephrotoxicity between IOCM and LOCM, several specialty medical societies have published guidelines on this issue (Table 3). Overall, these guidelines do not favor the use of IOCM over LOCM in high-risk patients.

SUMMARY

HOCM have been eliminated from procedural or diagnostic use requiring intravascular/intraarterial CM. In patients at high risk for CIN, despite the hope that IOCM would be less nephrotoxic than LOCM in a manner in which LOCM were found to be less nephrotoxic than HOCM and despite initial studies that supported a reduced nephrotoxicity with IOCM, subsequent clinical and experimental studies for the most part have failed to demonstrate reduced nephrotoxicity with IOCM. As such, multiple professional society guidelines do not favor IOCM over LOCM in high-risk patients for CIN. The authors of this article prefer LOCM over IOCM due to equivalent nephrotoxicity risk and reduced cost of LOCM.

There is newer literature emerging on renal-safe CM. One such example is adding the substituted cyclodextrin, sulfobutyl-ether-β-cyclodextrin, to iohexol in rodent models of nephrotoxicity to minimize toxicity.[109] The authors eagerly wait for newer agents that do not have the same nephrotoxic effect as current agents, especially in the high-risk patient population.

DISCLOSURE

The authors have nothing to disclose.

REFERENCES

1. Almen T. Visipaque–a step forward. A historical review. Acta Radiol Suppl 1995;399:2–18.
2. Almen T. Visipaque - a step forward: a historical review. Acta Radiol 2016;57(5):e47–63.
3. Haschek E, Lindenthal OT. A contribution to the practical use of the photography according to Röntgen. Wien Klin Wochenschr 1896;9:63.
4. Quader MA, Sawmiller CJ, Sumpio BE. Radio contrast agents: history and evolution. In: Chang JB, editor. Textbook of angiology. New York: Springer New York; 2000. p. 775–83.
5. Frank O, Alwens W. Kreislaufstudien am rontgenschirm. Munch Med Wochenschr 1910;57:950.
6. Berberich J, Hirsch S. Die röntgenographische Darstellung der Arterien und Venen am lebenden Menschen. J Mol Med 1923;2(49):2226–8.
7. Cameron DF. Aqueous solutions of potassium and sodium iodids as opaque mediums in roentgenography: preliminary report. J Am Med Assoc 1918;70(11):754–5.
8. Osborne ED, Sutherland CG, Scholl AJ, et al. Roentgenography of urinary tract during excretion of sodium iodide. J Am Med Assoc 1923; 80(6):368–73.
9. Binz A, Rath Ct. Uber biochemische Eigenschaften von Derivaten des Pyridins und Chinolins. Biochem Z 1928;203(218):16–103.
10. Swick M. Darstellung der Niere und Harnwege im Röntgenbild durch intravenöse Einbringung eines neuen Kontraststoffes, des Uroselectans. J Mol Med 1929;8(45):2087–9.
11. Hoey GB, Wiegert PE, Rands R. Organic iodine compounds as X-ray contrast media, vol. 76. Oxford (England): Pergamon Press; 1971.
12. Wallingford VH. The development of organic iodine compounds as x-ray contrast media. J Am Pharm Assoc Am Pharm Assoc 1953;42(12): 721–8.
13. Buschur M, Aspelin P. Contrast media: history and chemical properties. Interv Cardiol Clin 2014;3(3): 333–9.
14. Sovak M. Contrast media: a journey almost sentimental. Invest Radiol 1994;29(Suppl 1):S4–14.
15. Zamora CA, Castillo M. Historical perspective of imaging contrast agents. Magn Reson Imaging Clin N Am 2017;25(4):685–96.
16. Almen T. Contrast agent design. Some aspects on the synthesis of water soluble contrast agents of low osmolality. J Theor Biol 1969;24(2):216–26.
17. McClennan BL. Low-osmolality contrast media: premises and promises. Radiology 1987;162(1 Pt 1):1–8.
18. National Center for Biotechnology Information. PubChem Database. Diatrizoic acid C. Available at: https://pubchem.ncbi.nlm.nih.gov/compound/Diatrizoic-acid. Accessed October 27, 2019.
19. Almen T, Boijsen E, Lindell SE. Metrizamide in angiography I. Femoral angiography. Acta Radiol Diagn 1977;18(1):33–8.
20. Thomsen HS, Morcos SK. Radiographic contrast media. BJU Int 2000;86(Suppl 1):1–10.
21. Aspelin P. Contrast media: safety issues and ESUR guidelines. Springer Science & Business Media; 2009.
22. GE Healthcare Ireland, Cork, Ireland. Omnipaque (Iohexol). Silver Spring (MD): U.S. Food and Drug Administration; 2017. Available at: https://www.accessdata.fda.gov/drugsatfda_docs/nda/pre96/018956-s28_omnipaque_toc.cfm. Accessed January 14, 2020.

23. Sterling KA, Tehrani T, Rudnick MR. Clinical significance and preventive strategies for contrast-induced nephropathy. Curr Opin Nephrol Hypertens 2008;17(6):616–23.

24. Seeliger E, Flemming B, Wronski T, et al. Viscosity of contrast media perturbs renal hemodynamics. J Am Soc Nephrol 2007;18(11):2912–20.

25. GE Healthcare Ireland, Cork, Ireland. VISIPAQUE (iodixanol) injection. Silver Spring (MD): U.S. Food and Drug Administration Website; 2017. Available at: https://www.accessdata.fda.gov/drugsatfda_docs/label/2017/020808s026lbl.pdf. Accessed January 13, 2020.

26. Dawson P, Cosgrove DO, Grainger RG. Textbook of contrast media. Radiology 2000;217(1):138.

27. Bartels ED, Brun GC, Gammeltoft A, et al. Acute anuria following intravenous pyelography in a patient with myelomatosis. Acta Med Scand 1954; 150:297–302.

28. ACR manual on contast media. 11th edition. ACR.ACR Committee on Drugs and Contast; 2018.

29. McCullough PA, Wolyn R, Rocher LL, et al. Acute renal failure after coronary intervention: incidence, risk factors, and relationship to mortality. Am J Med 1997;103(5):368–75.

30. Rudnick M, Feldman H. Contrast-induced nephropathy: what are the true clinical consequences? Clin J Am Soc Nephrol 2008;3(1):263–72.

31. Spataro RF. Newer contrast agents for urography. Radiol Clin North Am 1984;22(2):365–80.

32. Brezis M, Rosen S. Hypoxia of the renal medulla–its implications for disease. N Engl J Med 1995; 332(10):647–55.

33. Heyman SN, Rosen S, Brezis M. Radiocontrast nephropathy: a paradigm for the synergism between toxic and hypoxic insults in the kidney. Exp Nephrol 1994;2(3):153–7.

34. Rudnick MR, Goldfarb S. Pathogenesis of contrast-induced nephropathy: experimental and clinical observations with an emphasis on the role of osmolality. Rev Cardiovasc Med 2003; 4(Suppl 5):S28–33.

35. Barrett BJ, Carlisle EJ. Metaanalysis of the relative nephrotoxicity of high- and low-osmolality iodinated contrast media. Radiology 1993;188(1):171–8.

36. McClennan BL, Stolberg HO. Intravascular contrast media. Ionic versus nonionic: current status. Radiol Clin North Am 1991;29(3):437–54.

37. Golman K, Almen T. Contrast media-induced nephrotoxicity. Survey and present state. Invest Radiol 1985;20(1 Suppl):S92–7.

38. Russell SB, Sherwood T. Monomer-dimer contrast media in the renal circulation: experimental angiography. Br J Radiol 1974;47(557):268–71.

39. Morris TW, Katzberg RW, Fischer HW. A comparison of the hemodynamic responses to metrizamide and meglumine/sodium diatrizoate in canine renal angiography. Invest Radiol 1978; 13(1):74–8.

40. Lund G, Rysavy J, Salomonowitz E, et al. Nephrotoxicity of contrast media assessed by occlusion arteriography. Radiology 1984;152(3):615–9.

41. Tornquist C, Almen T, Golman K, et al. Renal function following nephroangiography with metrizamide and iohexol. Effects on renal blood flow, glomerular permeability and filtration rate and diuresis in dogs. Acta Radiol Diagn 1985;26(4):483–9.

42. Katzberg RW, Morris TW, Lasser EC, et al. Acute systemic and renal hemodynamic effects of meglumine/sodium diatrizoate 76% and iopamidol in euvolemic and dehydrated dogs. Invest Radiol 1986;21(10):793–7.

43. Deray G, Baumelou B, Martinez F, et al. Renal vasoconstriction after low and high osmolar contrast agents in ischemic and non ischemic canine kidney. Clin Nephrol 1991;36(2):93–6.

44. Holtas S, Billstrom A, Tejler L. Proteinuria following nephroangiography. IX. Chemical and morphological analysis in dogs. Acta Radiol Diagn 1981;22(4):427–33.

45. Thomsen HS, Hemmingsen L, Golman K, et al. Low sodium diet, indomethacin, and contrast media. A comparison between renal effects of diatrizoate and iohexol in rats. Acta Radiol 1990;31(6):613–8.

46. Thomsen HS, Dorph S, Mygind T, et al. Urine profiles following intravenous diatrizoate, iohexol, or ioxilan in rats. Invest Radiol 1988;23(Suppl 1):S168–70.

47. Deray G, Dubois M, Martinez F, et al. Renal effects of radiocontrast agents in rats: a new model of acute renal failure. Am J Nephrol 1990;10(6):507–13.

48. Messana JM, Cieslinski DA, Nguyen VD, et al. Comparison of the toxicity of the radiocontrast agents, iopamidol and diatrizoate, to rabbit renal proximal tubule cells in vitro. J Pharmacol Exp Ther 1988;244(3):1139–44.

49. Rudnick MR, Berns JS, Cohen RM, et al. Nephrotoxic risks of renal angiography: contrast media-associated nephrotoxicity and atheroembolism–a critical review. Am J Kidney Dis 1994;24(4):713–27.

50. Gomes AS, Lois JF, Baker JD, et al. Acute renal dysfunction in high-risk patients after angiography: comparison of ionic and nonionic contrast media. Radiology 1989;170(1 Pt 1):65–8.

51. Schwab SJ, Hlatky MA, Pieper KS, et al. Contrast nephrotoxicity: a randomized controlled trial of a nonionic and an ionic radiographic contrast agent. N Engl J Med 1989;320(3):149–53.

52. Parfrey PS, Griffiths SM, Barrett BJ, et al. Contrast material-induced renal failure in patients with

diabetes mellitus, renal insufficiency, or both. A prospective controlled study. N Engl J Med 1989;320(3):143–9.

53. Harris KG, Smith TP, Cragg AH, et al. Nephrotoxicity from contrast material in renal insufficiency: ionic versus nonionic agents. Radiology 1991;179(3):849–52.

54. Taliercio CP, Vlietstra RE, Ilstrup DM, et al. A randomized comparison of the nephrotoxicity of iopamidol and diatrizoate in high risk patients undergoing cardiac angiography. J Am Coll Cardiol 1991;17(2):384–90.

55. Barrett BJ, Parfrey PS, Vavasour HM, et al. Contrast nephropathy in patients with impaired renal function: high versus low osmolar media. Kidney Int 1992;41(5):1274–9.

56. Moore RD, Steinberg EP, Powe NR, et al. Nephrotoxicity of high-osmolality versus low-osmolality contrast media: randomized clinical trial. Radiology 1992;182(3):649–55.

57. Rudnick MR, Goldfarb S, Wexler L, et al. Nephrotoxicity of ionic and nonionic contrast media in 1196 patients: a randomized trial. The Iohexol Cooperative Study. Kidney Int 1995;47(1):254–61.

58. Berg KJ. Nephrotoxicity related to contrast media. Scand J Urol Nephrol 2000;34(5):317–22.

59. Rudnick MR, Davidson C, Laskey W, et al. Nephrotoxicity of iodixanol versus ioversol in patients with chronic kidney disease: the Visipaque Angiography/Interventions with Laboratory Outcomes in Renal Insufficiency (VALOR) Trial. Am Heart J 2008;156(4):776–82.

60. Lautin EM, Freeman NJ, Schoenfeld AH, et al. Radiocontrast-associated renal dysfunction: a comparison of lower-osmolality and conventional high-osmolality contrast media. AJR Am J Roentgenol 1991;157(1):59–65.

61. Rihal CS, Textor SC, Grill DE, et al. Incidence and prognostic importance of acute renal failure after percutaneous coronary intervention. Circulation 2002;105(19):2259–64.

62. Cochran ST, Wong WS, Roe DJ. Predicting angiography-induced acute renal function impairment: clinical risk model. AJR Am J Roentgenol 1983;141(5):1027–33.

63. Manske CL, Sprafka JM, Strony JT, et al. Contrast nephropathy in azotemic diabetic patients undergoing coronary angiography. Am J Med 1990;89(5):615–20.

64. Morcos SK. Contrast media-induced nephrotoxicity—questions and answers. Br J Radiol 1998;71(844):357–65.

65. Weisberg LS, Kurnik PB, Kurnik BR. Risk of radiocontrast nephropathy in patients with and without diabetes mellitus. Kidney Int 1994;45(1):259–65.

66. Eng J, Wilson RF, Subramaniam RM, et al. Comparative effect of contrast media type on the incidence of contrast-induced nephropathy: a systematic review and meta-analysis. Ann Intern Med 2016;164(6):417–24.

67. Premawardhana D, Sekar B, Ul-Haq MZ, et al. Routine iso-osmolar contrast media use and acute kidney injury following percutaneous coronary intervention for ST elevation myocardial infarction. Minerva Cardioangiol 2019;67(5):380–91.

68. Barrett BJ, Katzberg RW, Thomsen HS, et al. Contrast-induced nephropathy in patients with chronic kidney disease undergoing computed tomography: a double-blind comparison of iodixanol and iopamidol. Invest Radiol 2006;41(11):815–21.

69. Carraro M, Malalan F, Antonione R, et al. Effects of a dimeric vs a monomeric nonionic contrast medium on renal function in patients with mild to moderate renal insufficiency: a double-blind, randomized clinical trial. Eur Radiol 1998;8(1):144–7.

70. Grynne BH, Nossen JO, Bolstad B, et al. Main results of the first comparative clinical studies on Visipaque. Acta Radiol Suppl 1995;399:265–70.

71. Murakami R, Tajima H, Kumazaki T, et al. Effect of iodixanol on renal function immediately after abdominal angiography. Clinical comparison with iomeprol and ioxaglate. Acta Radiol 1998;39(4):368–71.

72. Jakobsen JA, Berg KJ, Kjaersgaard P, et al. Angiography with nonionic X-ray contrast media in severe chronic renal failure: renal function and contrast retention. Nephron 1996;73(4):549–56.

73. McCullough PA, Bertrand ME, Brinker JA, et al. A meta-analysis of the renal safety of isosmolar iodixanol compared with low-osmolar contrast media. J Am Coll Cardiol 2006;48(4):692–9.

74. Solomon R. The role of osmolality in the incidence of contrast-induced nephropathy: a systematic review of angiographic contrast media in high risk patients. Kidney Int 2005;68(5):2256–63.

75. Heinrich MC, Haberle L, Muller V, et al. Nephrotoxicity of iso-osmolar iodixanol compared with nonionic low-osmolar contrast media: meta-analysis of randomized controlled trials. Radiology 2009;250(1):68–86.

76. Reed M, Meier P, Tamhane UU, et al. The relative renal safety of iodixanol compared with low-osmolar contrast media: a meta-analysis of randomized controlled trials. JACC Cardiovasc Interv 2009;2(7):645–54.

77. From AM, Al Badarin FJ, McDonald FS, et al. Iodixanol versus low-osmolar contrast media for prevention of contrast induced nephropathy: meta-analysis of randomized, controlled trials. Circ Cardiovasc Interv 2010;3(4):351–8.

78. Biondi-Zoccai G, Lotrionte M, Thomsen HS, et al. Nephropathy after administration of iso-osmolar and low-osmolar contrast media: evidence from a network meta-analysis. Int J Cardiol 2014; 172(2):375–80.

79. McCullough PA, Brown JR. Effects of intra-arterial and intravenous iso-osmolar contrast medium (iodixanol) on the risk of contrast-induced acute kidney injury: a meta-analysis. Cardiorenal Med 2011;1(4):220–34.

80. Dong M, Jiao Z, Liu T, et al. Effect of administration route on the renal safety of contrast agents: a meta-analysis of randomized controlled trials. J Nephrol 2012;25(3):290–301.

81. Sharma SK, Kini A. Effect of nonionic radiocontrast agents on the occurrence of contrast-induced nephropathy in patients with mild-moderate chronic renal insufficiency: pooled analysis of the randomized trials. Catheter Cardiovasc Interv 2005;65(3):386–93.

82. Zhang BC, Wu Q, Wang C, et al. A meta-analysis of the risk of total cardiovascular events of iso-smolar iodixanol compared with low-osmolar contrast media. J Cardiol 2014;63(4):260–8.

83. Zhang J, Jiang Y, Rui Q, et al. Iodixanol versus iopromide in patients with renal insufficiency undergoing coronary angiography with or without PCI. Medicine 2018;97(18):e0617.

84. Han XF, Zhang XX, Liu KM, et al. Contrast-induced nephropathy in patients with diabetes mellitus between iso- and low-osmolar contrast media: a meta-analysis of full-text prospective, randomized controlled trials. PLoS One 2018; 13(3):e0194330.

85. Zhao F, Lei R, Yang SK, et al. Comparative effect of iso-osmolar versus low-osmolar contrast media on the incidence of contrast-induced acute kidney injury in diabetic patients: a systematic review and meta-analysis. Cancer Imaging 2019; 19(1):38.

86. Aspelin P, Aubry P, Fransson SG, et al. Nephrotoxic effects in high-risk patients undergoing angiography. N Engl J Med 2003;348(6):491–9.

87. Laskey W, Aspelin P, Davidson C, et al. Nephrotoxicity of iodixanol versus iopamidol in patients with chronic kidney disease and diabetes mellitus undergoing coronary angiographic procedures. Am Heart J 2009;158(5):822–8.e3.

88. Solomon RJ, Natarajan MK, Doucet S, et al. Cardiac Angiography in Renally Impaired Patients (CARE) study: a randomized double-blind trial of contrast-induced nephropathy in patients with chronic kidney disease. Circulation 2007;115(25):3189–96.

89. Dillman JR, al-Hawary M, Ellis JH, et al. Comparative investigation of i.v. iohexol and iopamidol: effect on renal function in low-risk outpatients

undergoing CT. AJR Am J Roentgenol 2012; 198(2):392–7.

90. Becker J, Babb J, Serrano M. Glomerular filtration rate in evaluation of the effect of iodinated contrast media on renal function. AJR Am J Roentgenol 2013;200(4):822–6.

91. Koutsikos D, Konstadinidou I, Mourikis D, et al. Contrast media nephrotoxicity: comparison of diatrizoate, ioxaglate, and iohexol after intravenous and renal arterial administration. Ren Fail 1992;14(4):545–54.

92. Campbell DR, Flemming BK, Mason WF, et al. A comparative study of the nephrotoxicity of iohexol, iopamidol and ioxaglate in peripheral angiography. Can Assoc Radiol J 1990;41(3): 133–7.

93. Jevnikar AM, Finnie KJ, Dennis B, et al. Nephrotoxicity of high- and low-osmolality contrast media. Nephron 1988;48(4):300–5.

94. Heyman SN, Reichman J, Brezis M. Pathophysiology of radiocontrast nephropathy: a role for medullary hypoxia. Invest Radiol 1999;34(11): 685–91.

95. Deray G, Bagnis C, Jacquiaud C, et al. Renal effects of low and isoosmolar contrast media on renal hemodynamic in a normal and ischemic dog kidney. Invest Radiol 1999; 34(1):1–4.

96. Lancelot E, Idee JM, Lacledere C, et al. Effects of two dimeric iodinated contrast media on renal medullary blood perfusion and oxygenation in dogs. Invest Radiol 2002;37(7):368–75.

97. Ueda J, Nygren A, Hansell P, et al. Influence of contrast media on single nephron glomerular filtration rate in rat kidney. A comparison between diatrizoate, iohexol, ioxaglate, and iotrolan. Acta Radiol 1992;33(6):596–9.

98. Sendeski M, Patzak A, Pallone TL, et al. Iodixanol, constriction of medullary descending vasa recta, and risk for contrast medium-induced nephropathy. Radiology 2009;251(3):697–704.

99. Seeliger E, Becker K, Ladwig M, et al. Up to 50-fold increase in urine viscosity with iso-osmolar contrast media in the rat. Radiology 2010;256(2): 406–14.

100. Haneder S, Augustin J, Jost G, et al. Impact of iso- and low-osmolar iodinated contrast agents on BOLD and diffusion MRI in swine kidneys. Invest Radiol 2012;47(5):299–305.

101. Li LP, Lu J, Zhou Y, et al. Evaluation of intrarenal oxygenation in iodinated contrast-induced acute kidney injury-susceptible rats by blood oxygen level-dependent magnetic resonance imaging. Invest Radiol 2014;49(6):403–10.

102. Li LP, Lu J, Franklin T, et al. Effect of iodinated contrast medium in diabetic rat kidneys as evaluated by blood-oxygenation-level-dependent

magnetic resonance imaging and urinary neutrophil gelatinase-associated lipocalin. Invest Radiol 2015;50(6):392–6.

103. Wang YC, Tang A, Chang D, et al. Significant perturbation in renal functional magnetic resonance imaging parameters and contrast retention for iodixanol compared with iopromide: an experimental study using blood-oxygen-level-dependent/diffusion-weighted magnetic resonance imaging and computed tomography in rats. Invest Radiol 2014;49(11):699–706.

104. Liu TQ, Luo WL, Tan X, et al. A novel contrast-induced acute kidney injury model based on the 5/6-nephrectomy rat and nephrotoxicological evaluation of iohexol and iodixanol in vivo. Oxid Med Cell Longev 2014;2014:427560.

105. Cheng W, Zhao F, Tang CY, et al. Comparison of iohexol and iodixanol induced nephrotoxicity, mitochondrial damage and mitophagy in a new contrast-induced acute kidney injury rat model. Arch Toxicol 2018;92(7):2245–57.

106. Jo SH, Youn TJ, Koo BK, et al. Renal toxicity evaluation and comparison between visipaque (iodixanol) and hexabrix (ioxaglate) in patients with renal insufficiency undergoing coronary angiography: the RECOVER study: a randomized controlled trial. J Am Coll Cardiol 2006;48(5):924–30.

107. Thomsen HS, Morcos SK, Erley CM, et al. The ACTIVE Trial: comparison of the effects on renal function of iomeprol-400 and iodixanol-320 in patients with chronic kidney disease undergoing abdominal computed tomography. Invest Radiol 2008;43(3):170–8.

108. Liss P, Persson PB, Hansell P, et al. Renal failure in 57 925 patients undergoing coronary procedures using iso-osmolar or low-osmolar contrast media. Kidney Int 2006;70(10):1811–7.

109. Rowe ES, Rowe VD, Biswas S, et al. Preclinical Studies of a Kidney Safe Iodinated Contrast Agent. J Neuroimaging 2016;26(5):511–8.

110. Chalmers N, Jackson RW. Comparison of iodixanol and iohexol in renal impairment. Br J Radiol 1999;72(859):701–3.

111. Kidney Disease: Improving Global Outcomes Acute Kidney Injury Work Group. KDIGO clinical practice guideline for acute kidney injury. Kidney Int Suppl 2012;2:1–138.

112. Kushner FG, Hand M, Smith SC Jr, et al. 2009 focused updates: ACC/AHA guidelines for the management of patients with ST-elevation myocardial infarction (updating the 2004 guideline and 2007 focused update) and ACC/AHA/SCAI guidelines on percutaneous coronary intervention (updating the 2005 guideline and 2007 focused update) a report of the American College of Cardiology Foundation/American Heart Association Task Force on Practice Guidelines. J Am Coll Cardiol 2009;54(23):2205–41.

113. Wright RS, Anderson JL, Adams CD, et al. 2011 ACCF/AHA Focused Update of the Guidelines for the Management of Patients With Unstable Angina/Non-ST-Elevation Myocardial Infarction (Updating the 2007 Guideline): a report of the American College of Cardiology Foundation/American Heart Association Task Force on Practice Guidelines. Circulation 2011;123(18):2022–60.

114. Stacul F, van der Molen AJ, Reimer P, et al. Contrast induced nephropathy: updated ESUR Contrast Media Safety Committee guidelines. Eur Radiol 2011;21(12):2527–41.

115. Rudnick M. Prevention of contrast nephropathy associated with angiography. In: Forman J, editor. UpToDate. Retrieved March 22, 2020. Available at: https://www.uptodate.com/contents/prevention-of-contrast-nephropathy-associated-with-angiography.

Pathophysiology of Contrast-Induced Acute Kidney Injury

Shweta Bansal, MBBS, MD*, Rahul N. Patel, MD

KEYWORDS

- Contrast media adverse effects • Contrast media toxicity • Contrast-induced nephropathy
- Contrast-induced acute kidney injury • Contrast-associated acute kidney injury

KEY POINTS

- The two key mechanisms in the pathophysiology of CI-AKI are direct cytotoxic effects and hemodynamics alterations resulting in renal hypoperfusion.
- Direct cytotoxic effects, mainly to tubular epithelial and endothelial cells are mediated by oxidative stress and hypoxia.
- Hemodynamic alterations occur as a result of vasoconstriction and indirectly via endothelial damage of peritubular vasa recta, by oxygen free radicals.
- Thus, these pathways of contrast-induced acute kidney injury enhance and support each other.
- The hemodynamic alteration, oxidative stress and endothelial dysfunction associated with age, diabetes, heart failure and chronic kidney disease make these populations very susceptible for contrast induced acute kidney injury.

INTRODUCTION

Contrast-induced acute kidney injury (CI-AKI), lately referred as contrast-associated AKI, refers to AKI after intravenous or intra-arterial administration of contrast media (CM), defined as an increase in plasma creatinine level by a factor of 1.5 times or more over the baseline value within 7 days after exposure to contrast medium, or a plasma creatinine level that has increased by at least 0.3 mg/dL over the baseline value within 48 hours after exposure to contrast medium, or a urinary volume of less than 0.5 mL/kg of body weight per hour that persists for at least 6 hours after exposure.[1] The pathophysiology of AKI in general is complex, and most of the understanding of this condition comes from animal studies. The two key mechanisms in the pathophysiology of CI-AKI are direct cytotoxic effects and hemodynamics alterations that results in reduced glomerular filtration rate from kidney hypoperfusion.[2] Multiple distinct but potentially interacting pathways are recognized involving alterations in the renal hemodynamics from vasoactive mediators and hyperviscosity resulting in ischemia/hypoxia, oxidative stress, and direct CM toxicity to tubular epithelial and endothelial cells.[3] This article reviews the pathophysiology of CI-AKI by describing and explaining these pathways.

DIRECT CONTRAST MEDIA TUBULAR CELL TOXICITY

CM are tri-iodinated benzene derivatives. Iodine, in its ionic (I^-), molecular (I_2), or hydrated H_2OI^+ form is an antiseptic agent capable of lysing bacterial walls owing to its oxidizing power. The iodine contained in all types of CM—high osmolar, low osmolar, and iso-osmolar—has a direct toxic effect on human cells, and in particular on renal tubular epithelial cells (vacuolization of tubular cells and osmotic nephrosis) and on endothelial cells. The exact pathophysiologic mechanism of this cytotoxicity remains

Division of Nephrology, UT Health at San Antonio, 7703 Floyd Curl Dr, MSC 7882, San Antonio, TX 78229, USA
* Corresponding author.
E-mail address: BansalS3@uthscsa.edu

Intervent Cardiol Clin 9 (2020) 293–298
https://doi.org/10.1016/j.iccl.2020.03.001

unknown; however, several potential mechanisms have been suggested. CM could act by directly stimulating the signaling pathways involved in apoptosis via an activation of caspase-3, caspase-9 and the bcl2 pathway,[4] and by causing redistribution of membrane proteins, DNA fragmentation, disruption of intercellular junctions, reduced cell proliferation, and altered mitochondrial function via dysregulating calcium.[5–7] Recently, overexpression of microRNA-188 has been shown to induce apoptosis by regulating the SRSF7 gene, which may serve as a potential drug target for CI-AKI intervention.[8]

In general, the toxic effects of high osmolar CM are more pronounced than the effects of low osmolar or iso-osmolar CM, but all types of CM have negative effects on cell cultures.[5,6] In animal studies, CM alone has rarely been shown to cause overt renal damage unless accompanied by additional damage and the most common additional insult is some kind of ischemia/hypoxia.[9]

Oxidative Stress and Hypoxia

The intrinsic toxicity of CM is further accentuated by additional insults exerted by CM, such as oxidative stress and hypoxia.[10] CM, by their strong oxidizing power stimulate the synthesis of oxygen free radicles and reactive oxygen species (ROS) that are toxic to endothelial and tubular epithelial cells. Oxygen free radicals are molecules that contain one or more unpaired electrons, such as superoxide (O_2^-) and hydroxyl radical (OH^-).[3,11] During successive reduction reactions, these highly reactive molecules are turned into water.[3] Less aggressively reacting molecules, such as H_2O_2, are called ROS.[3,11] In the pathophysiology of CI-AKI, these types of molecules play a key role, because they interact with the other pathways. Highly reactive molecules create an imbalance between oxidants and antioxidants intracellularly, in favor of the oxidants, affecting mitochondrial and nuclear DNA, membrane lipids, and cellular proteins.[10] ROS activate c-Jun N-terminal kinases and p38MAPK stress kinases, which contribute to the apoptosis and necrosis.[12] In addition, ROS induces an increase in the synthesis of endothelin, angiotensin II, adenosine, and thromboxane A2, and a reduction in the synthesis of vasodilative nitric oxide (NO). The vasa recta, peritubular capillaries and glomerular capillaries acquire a vasoconstriction phenotype, causing alteration of renal microcirculation and distal ischemia.[13] In contrast, ischemia leads to increased formation of oxygen free radicals and ROS, so both

processes enhance each other (Fig. 1). Thus, once formed during hypoxia and/or cellular injury and exceeding the cellular scavenging capacities, oxygen free radicals and ROS lead to ischemia/reperfusion injury, a combination of both hypoxia and oxidative damage.[10] Endothelial damage in peritubular capillaries by CM directly or through ROS can be an important driving force of the medullary hypoxia.

Notably the ability to accommodate oxidative injury decreases with age.[14,15] Furthermore, patients with chronic kidney disease and diabetes already have increased oxidative stress, vasoconstrictors, and endothelial dysfunction,[16] making elderly, diabetic, and patients with chronic kidney disease very susceptible to CI-AKI.

IMPAIRMENT OF RENAL HEMODYNAMICS

Besides renal microcirculation effects caused by cell toxicity and increased oxidative stress, CM also have a direct effect on the renal vasculature. Under physiologic resting conditions, 25% of the cardiac output is directed toward the kidneys. The greater part of cardiac output is directed toward the cortex, to optimize glomerular filtration and reabsorption of water and salts.[17] The medullary blood flow is low; 10% of the renal blood flow represents medullary flow.[18] Its function is to preserve osmotic gradients and enhance urinary concentration.[17] Under physiologic circumstances, oxygen partial pressure (Po_2) levels of the renal cortex are approximately 50 mm Hg, whereas Po_2 levels of the renal medulla can be as low as 20 mm Hg.[17,19] The most vulnerable part of hypoxic damage is the deeper portion of the outer medulla that contains the metabolically active thick ascending limbs of the loop of Henle. In this part of the tubular system, an osmotic gradient is generated by active reabsorption of sodium, a process that requires a relatively large amount of oxygen.[17] Blood flow to the renal medulla is derived from efferent arterioles of juxtamedullary glomeruli. At the corticomedullary junction, these efferent arterioles give rise to the so-called descending vasa recta (DVR). These DVR gradually form a capillary bed that penetrates deep into the inner medulla. These capillaries eventually coalesce to form the ascending vasa recta (Fig. 2). The transformation from DVR to capillaries and thence to the ascending vasa recta occurs gradually, with accompanying histologic changes in the composition of the vessel wall.[20] After intravascular administration, CM display a rapid distribution over intravascular and interstitial fluids. The distribution half-life is usually several

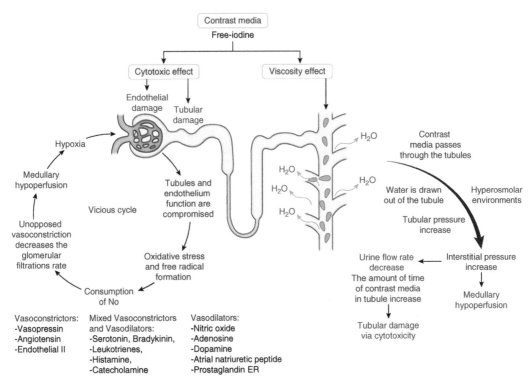

Fig. 1. The proposed mechanism of contrast-media-mediated nephrotoxicity. (*Adapted from* Morcos R, Kucharik M, Bansal P, et al. Contrast-induced acute kidney injury: review and practical update. Clinical Medicine Insights: Cardiology Volume 13: 1–9; with permission.)

minutes, ranging from 2 to 30 minutes. Only 1% to 3% is bound by plasma proteins.[21] CM are not metabolized in humans, but are eliminated quickly through glomerular filtration by the kidneys. The elimination half-life, or time to clear one-half of the amount of CM in the blood, is approximately 1 to 2 hours.[21] In the first 24 hours after intravascular administration of CM, approximately 100% of the CM is excreted in the urine in patients with a normal renal function; however, this time can increase to 40 hours or more in patients with decreased renal function.[21] Alternative routes of elimination, such as biliary elimination, are slow. The hemodynamic response to intra-arterial injection of CM is biphasic: a brief initial increase in renal blood flow followed by a prolonged decline of 10% to 25% below baseline.[3,18,22] This process predominantly reflects a decrease in cortical blood flow, as 10% of renal blood flow represents medullary flow.[18] Decreases of outer medullary Po_2 by 50% to 67% after CM administration to 9 to 15 mm Hg have been reported.[11,18]

In recent years, several animal studies have gained more insight into the hemodynamic response of renal microvasculature, particularly DVR to CM. The average DVR diameter is 12

to 18 mm, close to that of a red blood cell. On isolated rat DVRs, it has been shown that microperfusion with iodixanol leads to a diameter reduction of 48%, caused by a decrease in NO production and an increase in reactivity of DVR to angiotensin II. The addition of a free radical scavenger prevented vasoconstriction induced by iodixanol and angiotensin II.[23]

Additionally, decreased NO availability and increased superoxide production also result in a pronounced vasoconstrictive effect on afferent arterioles than on efferent arterioles after CM administration in isolated mouse kidney vessels.[24] Moreover, perfusion of human and rat renal arteries (interlobar) with CM has shown to cause endothelial cell damage and increased endothelial permeability. It was postulated that DVR constriction is a consequence of endothelial damage and decreased NO avalaibility.[13] Along the same concept, pretreatment of animals with phosphodiesterase type 5 inhibitor, which increases NO availability, or nitrite infusion was associated with lesser degree of histologic injury and attenuation in markers of AKI.[25–27] To summarize, these experiments suggest that administration of CM decreases NO availability via endothelial damage and leads to

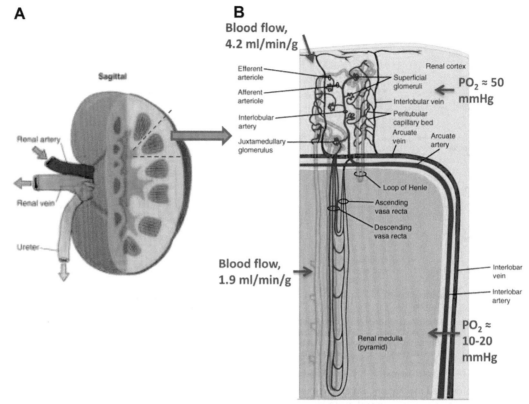

Fig. 2. (*A, B*) Anatomy of vascularization and (patho)physiology of medulla. The PO$_2$ of the cortex is approximately 50 mm Hg and decreases to 25 mm Hg after CM administration. The PO$_2$ of the medulla is approximately 20 mm Hg, and decreases to 9 to 15 mm Hg after CM administration. The most vulnerable part for ischemia is the thick ascending limb from the loop of Henle in the outer medulla. ([*A*] *From* Costanzo L. Physiology. 6th ed. Elsevier; 2017, Chapter 6; [*B*] *From* Boron W, Boulpaep E. Medical Physiology. 3rd ed. Elsevier; 2016, Chapter 33; with permission.)

vasoconstriction of afferent arteriole and thus the glomerular filtration rate; and promote direct cell toxicity as a result of hypoxia from medullary DVR vasoconstriction. In addition to NO and angiotensin, multiple other vasoactive mediators play a crucial role in the decrease in regional blood flow after CM administration. Prominent medullary vasodilators include adenosine, dopamine, NO, atrial natriuretic peptide, and prostaglandin E2.[17,19,22] Potent vasoconstrictors include vasopressin, angiotensin II, and endothelin.[17–19] Potential additional participants, with both dilative and constrictive properties, are serotonin, bradykinin, leukotrienes, histamine, and catecholamines.[22] It is unknown as to what extent each mediator plays a role in the pathogenesis of CI-AKI, but an imbalance occurs between vasoconstrictive and vasodilative mediators in favor of the vasoconstrictive mediators. Furthermore, the distribution of receptor mediator subtypes in the cortex and medulla may be responsible for different regional hemodynamic responses[18,22] (see **Fig. 1**). Because these studies have been conducted with iodixanol as the agent

investigated, it would be interesting to repeat these experiments with a low osmolar CM. The only additional study published in this area of research compared the effect on DVR constriction of the high-osmolar ionic CM amidotrizoate with the low osmolar ioxaglate, the low osmolar iopromide, and the iso-osmolar iodixanol.[28] All 4 types of CM showed DVR constriction rates between 45% and 63% and these differences were not statistically significant.[28]

With advancing age, there is a decrease in renal plasma flow as well the glomerular filtration rate and a significant decrease in the capillary ultrafiltration coefficient as a result of the decreases in both the glomerular capillary permeability and the surface area availability for filtration.[29,30] Similarly, patients with heart failure have a decreased renal blood flow and glomerular filtration rate as a result of neurohormomal activation and inflammation.[31] As a consequence, elderly patients with heart failure are at an increased risk of CI-AKI given their already compromised renal blood flow.

As described elsewhere in this article, a decrease in regional microcirculatory blood flow ensues into medullary hypoxia, which is further exacerbated by increased oxygen demand of tubular cells.[11,18] This increased oxygen demand of the tubular cells is a phenomenon that occurs after injection of CM with an osmolality higher than blood (ie, high osmolar or low osmolar CM), which leads to a transient increase in renal plasma flow, glomerular filtration rate, and urinary output.[18] Because of both osmotic load and the effect of endothelin release, more sodium has to be reabsorbed by distal tubular cells,[11,18,19] which leads to increased oxygen consumption.[19,22] This effect is virtually nonexistent in iso-osmolar CM, a theoretic advantage of this type of CM. In contrast, a decrease in contact time between the CM and renal tubular cells as a result of increased renal plasma flow, glomerular filtration, and urinary output represent a theoretic advantage of high osmolar and low osmolar CM over iso-osmolar CM. Moreover, iso-osmolar CM have a higher viscosity than low osmolar CM, with comparable iodine concentrations, which has been associated with increased amount and period of time of iodine retention by the kidney, cell injury, and expression of kidney injury markers in animal studies. Furthermore, a decrease in renal blood oxygen levels and an increased formation of vacuoles in the renal tubular epithelium of the cortex, predominantly in the proximal and distal tubules, have been shown.[32,33] Nevertheless, these risks and advantages have been more theoretic; in clinical studies, there are not many differences in incidence of CI-AKI with iso-osmolar versus low osmolar CM.[34]

SUMMARY

The passage of CM through the renal vascular bed leads to vasoconstriction. The perfusion decrease in the physiologically poorly oxygenated medulla leads to ischemia of tubular cells. Through both ischemia and direct toxicity to renal tubular cells, ROS formation is increased, which enhances the effect of vasoconstrictive mediators and decreases the bioavailability of vasodilative mediators. Furthermore, ROS formation leads to oxidative damage to tubular cells. These three interacting pathways, namely, hemodynamic effects, an increase in oxygen free radicals, and direct CM molecule tubular cell toxicity, lead to tubular necrosis. The preexistent risk factors such as advance age, heart failure, chronic kidney disease, and diabetes associated with decreased renal blood flow, altered vasoactive mediators, and increased oxidative stress further compound these pathophysiologic mechanisms and make these patients very susceptible to CI-AKI. In the pathophysiology of CI-AKI, two types of frequently used CM—low osmolar and iso-osmolar—have their theoretic advantages and disadvantages related to their hyperosmolarity and hyperviscocity, respectively, relative to blood; however, clinically the difference in incidence of CI-AKI has not been evident.

REFERENCES

1. KDIGO Clinical practice guideline for acute kidney injury. Kidney Int Suppl 2012;2:1–138.
2. Bellomo R, Kellum JA, Ronco C. Acute kidney injury. Lancet 2012;380:756–66.
3. Katzberg RW. Contrast medium-induced nephrotoxicity; which pathway? Radiology 2005;235:752–5.
4. Romano G, Briguori C, Quintavalle C, et al. Contrast agent and renal cell apoptosis. Eur Heart J 2008;29(20):2569–76.
5. Haller C, Hizoh I. The cytotoxicity of iodinated radiocontrast agents on renal cells in vitro. Invest Radiol 2004;39:149–54.
6. Sendeski MM. Pathophysiology of renal tissue damage by iodinated contrast media. Clin Exp Pharmacol Physiol 2011;38:292–9.
7. Ward DB, Brown KC, Valentovic MA. Radiocontrast agent diatrizoic acid induces mitophagy and oxidative stress via calcium dysregulation. Int J Mol Sci 2019;20(17) [pii:E4074].
8. Liu B, Chai Y, Guo W. MicroRNA-188 aggravates contrast-induced apoptosis by targeting SRSF7 in novel isotonic contrast-induced acute kidney injury rat models and renal tubular epithelial cells. Ann Transl Med 2019;7(16):378.
9. Kiss N, Hamar P. Histopathological evaluation of contrast-induced acute kidney injury rodent models. Biomed Res Int 2016;2016:3763250.
10. Heyman SN, Rosen S, Khamaisi M, et al. Reactive oxygen species and the pathogenesis of radiocontrast-induced nephropathy. Invest Radiol 2010;45:188–95.
11. Persson PB, Hansell P, Liss P. Pathophysiology of contrast medium-induced nephropathy. Kidney Int 2005;68:14–22.
12. Briguori C, Donnarumma E, Quintavalle C, et al. Contrast induced acute kidney injury: potential new strategies. Curr Opin Nephrol Hypertens 2015;24:145–53.
13. Sendeski MM, Persson AB, Liu ZZ, et al. Iodinated contrast media cause endothelial damage leading to vasoconstriction of human and rat vasa recta. Am J Physiol Renal Physiol 2012;303: 1592–8.

14. Baylis C. Sexual dimorphism in the aging kidney: differences in the nitric oxide system. Nat Rev Nephrol 2009;5:384–96.

15. Delp MD, Behnke BJ, Spier SA, et al. Ageing diminishes endothelium-dependent vasodilatation and tetrahydrobiopterin content in rat skeletal muscle arterioles. J Physiol 2008;586:1161–8.

16. Heyman SN, Rosenberger C, Rosen S, et al. Why is diabetes mellitus a risk factor for contrast-induced nephropathy? Biomed Res Int 2013;2013:123589.

17. Brezis M, Rosen S. Hypoxia of the renal medulla—its implications for disease. N Engl J Med 1995;332: 647–55.

18. Heyman SN, Rosen S, Rosenberger C. Renal parenchymal hypoxia, hypoxia adaptation and the pathogenesis of radiocontrast nephropathy. Clin J Am Soc Nephrol 2008;3:288–96.

19. Heyman SN, Reichman J, Brezis M. Pathophysiology of radiocontrast nephropathy. Invest Radiol 1999;34:685–91.

20. Pallone TL, Turner MR, Edwards A, et al. Countercurrent exchange in the renal medulla. Am J Physiol Regul Integr Comp Physiol 2003;284:R1153–75.

21. Speck U. Contrast media: overview, use and pharmaceutical aspects [corrected]. 4th edition. Berlin: Springer; 1999. p. 8–83.

22. Heyman SN, Rosenberger C, Rosen S. Regional alterations in renal hemodynamics and oxygenation: a role in contrast medium-induced nephropathy. Nephrol Dial Transplant 2005;20(Suppl 1):i6–11.

23. Sendeski M, Patzak A, Pallone T, et al. Iodixanol, constriction of medullary descending vasa recta, and risk for contrast medium-induced nephropathy. Radiology 2009;251:697–704.

24. Liu ZZ, Viegas VU, Perlewitx A, et al. Iodinated contrast media differentially affect afferent and efferent arteriolar tone and reactivity in mice: a possible explanation for reduced glomerular filtration rate. Radiology 2012;265:762–71.

25. Seeliger E, Cantow K, Arakelyan K, et al. Low-dose nitrite alleviates early effects of an X-ray contrast medium on renal hemodynamics and oxygenation in rats. Invest Radiol 2014;49:70–7.

26. Lauver DA, Carey EG, Bergin IL, et al. Sildenafil citrate for prophylaxis of nephropathy in an animal model of contrast-induced acute kidney injury. PLoS One 2014;9(11):e113598.

27. Armaly Z, Artol S, Jabbour AR, et al. Impact of pretreatment with carnitine and tadalafil on contrast-induced nephropathy in CKD patients. Ren Fail 2019;41(1):976–86.

28. Sendeski M, Patzak A, Persson PB. Constriction of the vasa recta, the vessels supplying the area at risk for acute kidney injury, by four different iodinated contrast media, evaluating ionic, non-ionic, monomeric and dimeric agents. Invest Radiol 2010;45:453–7.

29. Hoang K, Tan JC, Derby G, et al. Determinants of glomerular hypofiltration in aging humans. Kidney Int 2003;64:1417–24.

30. Weinstein JR, Anderson S. The aging kidney: physiological changes. Adv Chronic Kidney Dis 2010;17: 302–7.

31. Schrier RW. Role of diminished renal function in cardiovascular mortality: marker or pathogenetic factor? J Am Coll Cardiol 2006; 47(1):1–8.

32. Lenhard DC, Pietsch HM, Sieber MA, et al. The osmolality of non-ionic, iodinated contrast agents as an important factor for renal safety. Invest Radiol 2012;47:503–10.

33. Lenhard DC, Frisk AL, Lengsfeld P, et al. The effect of iodinated contrast agent properties on renal kinetics and oxygenation. Invest Radiol 2013;48:175–82.

34. Eng J, Wilson RF, Subramaniam RM, et al. Comparative effect of contrast media type on the incidence of contrast-induced nephropathy: a systematic review and meta-analysis. Ann Intern Med 2016;164(6):417–24.

Contrast-Induced Acute Kidney Injury—Definitions, Epidemiology, and Implications

Lorenzo Azzalini, MD, PhD, MSc[a],*, Sanjog Kalra, MD, MSc[b]

KEYWORDS

- Contrast-induced nephropathy • Contrast-induced acute kidney injury • Contrast media
- Epidemiology

KEY POINTS

- Contrast-induced acute kidney injury (CI-AKI) frequently is observed in patients undergoing a variety of catheter-based interventional procedures.
- Exact estimates and comparisons in the literature have traditionally been hampered by heterogeneous definitions.
- With the increasing complexity of patients undergoing coronary, endovascular, and structural interventions, the burden of CI-AKI is expected to increase.
- CI-AKI is associated with increased rates of short-term and long-term adverse events (including death) and, therefore, is linked to increased length of stay and health care costs.

INTRODUCTION

Contrast-induced acute kidney injury (CI-AKI) is the acute onset of renal injury after exposure to iodinated contrast media (CM) in a variety of diagnostic and interventional procedures, including catheter-based angiography and interventions.

The causal association between exposure to CM and development of acute kidney injury (AKI) has recently been questioned.[1–3] Studies linking CM exposure directly to kidney injury are confounded by both patient-related factors (age, chronic kidney disease [CKD], diabetes mellitus, and left ventricular dysfunction, among others) and procedure-related factors (eg, embolization of atheromatous material from the aorta during catheter manipulation, hypotension, and bleeding) that are independently associated with development of AKI.[4] Therefore, it might be more appropriate to utilize the term "contrast-associated AKI",[5] in acknowledgment of these causal uncertainties. Due to the solid body of experimental evidence on the toxic effects of CM at the tubular level,[4] however, as well as for historical reasons, this review maintains the term, "CI-AKI".

Contemporary definitions and diagnostic criteria set forth for CI-AKI are reviewed and the epidemiology and clinical implications of this condition discussed.

DEFINITIONS

The definition of CI-AKI has traditionally relied on serum creatinine (SCr), the most widely available marker of acute kidney disease and CKD. Several definitions have been used over the past decades and across different specialties, lending challenge to the estimation of the epidemiologic relevance of this condition and complicating comparisons in research.

Among the numerous definitions of CI-AKI (Table 1), the one set forth by the Kidney

[a] The Zena and Michael A. Wiener Cardiovascular Institute, Icahn School of Medicine at Mount Sinai, Klingenstein Clinical Center, 7th Floor North, 1450 Madison Avenue, New York, NY 10029, USA; [b] Einstein Heart and Vascular Institute, Einstein Medical Center Philadelphia, 5501 Old York Road, Philadelphia, PA 19085, USA
* Corresponding author.
E-mail address: lorenzo.azzalini@mountsinai.org
Twitter: @lorenzo2509 (L.A.)

Intervent Cardiol Clin 9 (2020) 299–309
https://doi.org/10.1016/j.iccl.2020.02.001
2211-7458/20/© 2020 Elsevier Inc. All rights reserved.

Table 1 Definitions of contrast-induced acute kidney injury	
Definition	**Author**
Increase of ≥0.5 mg/dL or ≥25% in SCr at 48 h	Mehran et al,[13] 2004
Increase of >0.5 mg/dL or >25% in SCr within 72 h	European Society of Urogenital Radiology[65]
Increase of ≥0.5 mg/dL from baseline	BMC2[20]

Increase of >50% in SCr or decrease of >25% in glomerular filtration rate or oliguria (<0.5 mL/kg/h for >6 h)
Stages
  Risk: SCr 1.5–2 times baseline or glomerular filtration rate decreased >25%; urinary volume <0.5 mL/kg/h for ≥6 h
  Injury: SCr 2–3 times baseline or glomerular filtration rate decreased >50%; urinary volume <0.5 mL/kg/h for ≥12 h
  Failure: SCr >3 times baseline or glomerular filtration rate decreased >75% or SCr ≥4 mg/dL with acute rise ≥0.5 mg/dL; urinary volume <0.3 mL/kg/h for ≥24 h or anuria for ≥12 h
  Loss of kidney function: persistent acute renal failure: complete loss of kidney function >4 wk (requiring dialysis)
  End-stage renal disease: complete loss of kidney function >3 mo (requiring dialysis)
	RIFLE[66]

Increase in SCr of ≥0.3 mg/dL or ≥50% from baseline or oliguria (<0.5 mL/kg/h for >6 h) within 48 h Stage 1: increase in SCr of ≥0.3 mg/dL or increase to ≥150% to 200% (1.5-fold to 2-fold) from baseline; urinary volume <0.5 mL/kg/h for >6 h Stage 2: increase in SCr to >200% to 300% (>2- to 3-fold) from baseline; urinary volume <0.5 mL/kg/h for >12 h Stage 3: increase in SCr to >300% (>3-fold) from baseline, SCr ≥4.0 mg/dL with an acute increase of >0.5 mg/dL; urinary volume <0.3 mL/kg/h for ≥24 h or anuria for ≥12 h	AKIN[15]
Increase in SCr of ≥1.5 times baseline within 7 d or increase in SCr by ≥0.3 mg/dL within 48 h or urinary volume of <0.5 mL/kg/h for ≥6 h Stage 1: SCr 1.5–1.9 times baseline or ≥0.3 mg/dL increase; urinary volume <0.5 mL/kg/h for ≥6 h Stage 2: SCr 2.0–2.9 times baseline; urinary volume <0.5 mL/kg/h for ≥12 h Stage 3: SCr ≥3 times baseline or increase in SCr to ≥4 mg/dL or initiation of renal replacement therapy; urinary volume <0.3 mL/kg/h for ≥24 h or anuria for ≥12 h	KDIGO[6]

Disease Improving Global Outcomes (KDIGO) initiative[6] is the most recent and incorporates key variables that allow it to capture the variety of clinical presentation patterns of CI-AKI: a low-grade but steady increase in SCr over the course of several days (≥1.5-times baseline within 7 days), a sudden increase in SCr within the immediate period after CM exposure (≥0.3 mg/dL within 48 h), and the development of oliguria (urinary volume of <0.5 mL/kg/h for ≥6 h). Moreover, it also provides a staging system, which makes it particularly useful to evaluate the clinical impact of a condition that has a tremendous variation in the severity of clinical presentation (from asymptomatic rise in SCr to clinically overt renal failure with need for urgent renal replacement therapy).

CI-AKI definitions based on alternative biomarkers have also been proposed. Cystatin C is more sensitive than sCr to rapidly detect acute changes in renal function.[7] Briguori and colleagues[8] identified an increase in serum cystatin C of greater than or equal to 10% above baseline at 24 hours after CM exposure as the optimal cutoff for the early identification of patients at risk for CI-AKI (negative predictive value 100% and positive predictive value 39.1%, utilizing an SCr increase of greater than or equal to 0.3 mg/dL within 48 h as the gold standard). Such CI-AKI definition also showed good correlation with 1-year outcomes. Another early biomarker of AKI that may be suitable for CI-AKI detection is neutrophil gelatinase–associated lipocalin. Quintavalle and colleagues[9] found that a serum neutrophil gelatinase–associated lipocalin value at 6 hours greater than or equal to 179 ng/mL had 93% negative predictive value and 20% positive predictive value for CI-AKI (defined by Briguori and colleagues[8]). At present, despite their potential interest, the utilization of these and other novel CI-AKI definitions based on alternative biomarkers is hampered by their limited availability and validation.

EPIDEMIOLOGY

Given the heterogeneity of CI-AKI definitions and the lack of systematic surveillance of SCr after CM-based diagnostic and interventional procedures, the wide range of CI-AKI incidences reported in the literature is not surprising. As such, a discussion about CI-AKI epidemiology classified by procedure type is presented, to facilitate understanding and application in clinical practice.

Coronary Angiography

It remains challenging to define the epidemiology of CI-AKI after coronary angiography, because most reports focus on patients mostly (or even exclusively) undergoing interventions. **Fig. 1** presents the incidence of CI-AKI across studies of coronary angiography.

The NEPHRIC trial[10] randomized 129 patients undergoing coronary or aortofemoral angiography with or without intervention to 1 of 2 iodinated CM: iodixanol or iohexol. CI-AKI, defined as an increase in SCr of greater than 0.5 mg/dL at 72 hours, was observed in 15%. Mean contrast volume used was quite high (approximately 160 mL), possibly reflecting older interventional cardiology practice, and 21% of patients in this study underwent

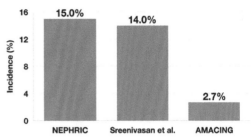

Fig. 1. Incidence of CI-AKI in coronary angiography studies.

intervention. Similarly, in a single-center retrospective study by Sreenivasan and colleagues,[11] CI-AKI (defined as an increase in SCr by ≥0.3 mg/dL within 48 h) was observed in 14%. Contrast volume used was 131 mL ± 89 mL (a much higher value than expected in a population of subjects exclusively undergoing coronary angiography, because only 34% of patients underwent concomitant PCI). Patients who did not have a postprocedural SCr value available were excluded from this study, which may have overestimated the true CI-AKI incidence. Finally, the AMACING trial,[12] which randomized 660 patients to undergo pre-CM exposure intravenous hydration versus no prophylaxis, included 48% of patients undergoing intra-arterial CM administration for coronary or peripheral angiography and only 16% of patients underwent interventions. The mean contrast volume administered was approximately 90 mL. Therefore, data from this trial can provide a reliable figure of CI-AKI incidence in patients undergoing contemporary diagnostic angiograms. CI-AKI, defined as an increase in SCr by greater than 25% or greater than 0.5 mg/dL within 2 to 6 days of CM exposure, was observed in only 2.7% of patients overall.

Percutaneous coronary intervention

A large amount of data is available on the epidemiology of CI-AKI in patients undergoing PCI (**Fig. 2A**). A seminal study by Mehran and colleagues[13] defined CI-AKI as an increase in SCr greater than or equal to 0.5 mg/dL or greater than or equal to 25% at 48 hours. This definition has since been used extensively in the literature. The incidence of CI-AKI in such study was 13.1%. In a recent single-center registry from the authors' group,[14] Acute Kidney Injury Network (AKIN)[15]-defined CI-AKI was observed in 11.7% of patients and CI-AKI requiring dialysis in 0.3%. In a meta-analysis of 36 randomized trials, including 7166 patients,[16] CI-AKI, defined as an increase in SCr greater than or equal to

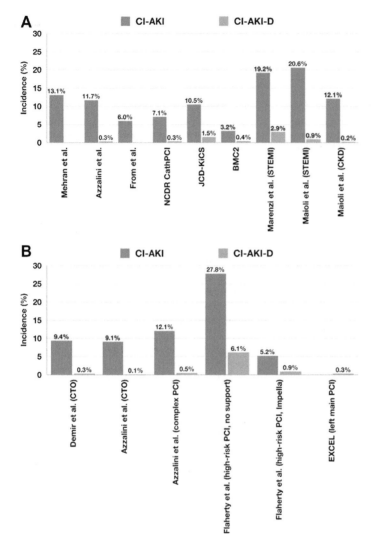

Fig. 2. Incidence of CI-AKI and CI-AKI requiring dialysis (CI-AKI-D) in studies of (A) all-comers undergoing PCI and (B) patients undergoing complex PCI.

0.5 mg/dL, was observed in 6.0%. When an alternative definition of an increase in SCr greater than 25% was used, the incidence rose to 9.0%. More contemporary data on the incidence of CI-AKI are available from studies utilizing large national registries. Data from the National Cardiovascular Disease Registry (NCDR) CathPCI Registry,[17] which included 985,737 consecutive patients undergoing percutaneous coronary intervention (PCI), indicate an overall incidence of AKIN-defined CI-AKI of 7.1% (stages 1, 2, and 3 AKI were diagnosed in 6.0%, 0.5%, and 0.3%, respectively), with 0.3% requiring initiation of dialysis. When the same definitions were applied to the Japan Cardiovascular Database–Keio interhospital Cardiovascular Studies (JCD-KiCS) registry,[18] the incidence rates of CI-AKI and CI-AKI requiring dialysis

were 10.5% and 1.5%, respectively. These higher figures might reflect differences in baseline characteristics of the study population, biological susceptibility to CI-AKI in the Japanese population, and/or practice patterns with regard to both PCI techniques and thresholds to initiate dialysis.[14] In an analysis from the Blue Cross Blue Shield of Michigan Cardiovascular Consortium (BMC2), Gurm and colleagues[19] observed incidence rates of CI-AKI and CI-AKI requiring dialysis of 3.2% and 0.4%, respectively. These lower rates can be traced to the CI-AKI definition used (increase in SCr ≥0.5 mg/dL during the week after PCI), which is less sensitive than definitions including lower absolute thresholds or relative changes.[20] Moreover, the increasing awareness of the association of CM volume with CI-AKI risk may have resulted in a change in practice toward using lower doses of CM for all patients undergoing PCI in Michigan.[21]

The incidence of CI-AKI is higher in reports focusing exclusively on patients with high-risk conditions. For example, acute coronary syndromes are associated with a systemic proinflammatory milieu and frequently hypotension. Marenzi and colleagues[22] reported an incidence of CI-AKI (increase in SCr >0.5 mg/dL) of 19.2% in patients undergoing primary PCI in the setting of ST-segment elevation myocardial infarction (STEMI) (2.9% required dialysis). Similar figures (20.6% and 0.9%, respectively) have been reported by others in this setting.[23] CKD is one of the strongest predictors of CI-AKI.[4,17] Maioli and colleagues[24] reported an incidence of CI-AKI (increase in SCr ≥0.5 mg/dL within 3 days) in 12.1% in patients with creatinine clearance less than 60 mL/min undergoing coronary angiography with or without intervention; new need for dialysis was observed in 0.2%. In the NCDR CathPCI Registry,[17] the incidence of AKIN-defined CI-AKI increased with decreasing estimated glomerular filtration rate (eGFR) categories from 5.2% in patients with an eGFR greater than or equal to 60 mL/min/1.73 m² to 26.6% in patients with an eGFR less than 30 mL/min/1.73 m². This was amplified in patients with STEMI (from 7.8% to 36.9%, respectively). The recent increase in patient-related and procedural complexity in the interventional cardiology arena has resulted in the recognition of a subset of patients who require percutaneous revascularization and are at higher risk for complications, including CI-AKI.[25] In this complex higher-risk (and indicated) patient (CHIP) subset, conditions predisposing to CI-AKI (advanced age, CKD, diabetes, decompensated heart failure, hemodynamic instability, use of aggressive PCI techniques, and so forth) are highly prevalent. A summary of the incidence of CI-AKI across studies in CHIP PCI cohorts is presented in Fig. 2B. Demir and colleagues[26] found no difference in AKIN-defined CI-AKI rates between patients undergoing chronic total occlusion (CTO) and non-CTO PCI (9.4% vs 12.1%; P = .17). This was confirmed in a sensitivity analysis including only patients who underwent CTO PCI in a stable clinical setting (7.7% vs 8.5%; P = .66) and on multivariable adjustment. In a multicenter study focusing exclusively on patients undergoing CTO PCI,[27] AKIN-defined CI-AKI incidence was 9.1% overall and was almost twice as high in CKD versus non-CKD patients (15.0% vs 7.8%; P = .001). The incidence of CI-AKI requiring dialysis followed a similar pattern

(0.5% vs 0%; P = .03). In another study from the authors' group,[28] there were no differences in the incidence of AKIN-defined CI-AKI and CI-AKI requiring dialysis in patients undergoing complex versus noncomplex PCI (12.1% vs 11.5%; P = .63 and 0.5% vs 0.2%; P = .25, respectively). Recently, Flaherty and colleagues[29] showed that the incidence of AKIN-defined (CI-)AKI and (CI-)AKI requiring dialysis is high in patients with severe left ventricular dysfunction undergoing high-risk PCI (27.8% and 6.1%, respectively). In this context, mechanical circulatory support as provided by Impella (Abiomed, Danvers, Massachusetts) is associated with a markedly lower risk of such complications (5.2% and 0.9%, respectively). Finally, in a subanalysis of the EXCEL trial, which assessed the outcomes of left main revascularization using PCI versus coronary artery bypass graft surgery, Giustino and colleagues[30] observed an incidence of acute renal failure (defined as SCr increase ≥5.0 mg/dL from baseline or new requirement for dialysis) and need for dialysis at 30 days of 0.6% and 0.3%, respectively, in patients undergoing left main PCI. Again, patients with CKD suffered a higher incidence of such complications (2.3% vs 0.3%, and 1.1% vs 0.1%, respectively).

Peripheral Interventions

Compared with the coronary space, relatively less literature is available to inform on the incidence of CI-AKI in peripheral angiography and intervention (Fig. 3). Patients undergoing such procedures usually suffer from extensive, polyvascular atherosclerotic disease and often present several CI-AKI risk factors (advanced age, diabetes, hypertension, and so forth). As such, these patients are at inherently higher risk for developing CI-AKI, for which peripheral arterial disease is considered a risk factor.[4] A study from the 1990s reported relatively low rates (6.9%) of CI-

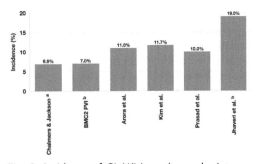

Fig. 3. Incidence of CI-AKI in endovascular intervention studies. [a] Only patients undergoing peripheral angiography. [b] Figures reported for the highest-risk groups.

AKI (defined as an increase in SCr >25% from baseline) in patients undergoing peripheral angiography and receiving on average approximately 55 mL of contrast.[31] Similarly, a report from the BMC2 Peripheral Vascular Intervention (BMC2 PVI) registry[32] on 7769 patients undergoing lower extremity peripheral interventions indicated an incidence of CI-AKI (increase in SCr ≥0.5 mg/dL) from 3% to 7% (increasing by age group). More contemporary studies, however, have challenged these findings. Arora and colleagues[33] reported an AKIN-defined CI-AKI incidence of 11% among patients undergoing endovascular therapy for chronic limb ischemia. Kim and colleagues,[34] who evaluated the incidence of Mehran-defined CI-AKI in patients undergoing endovascular therapy for intermittent claudication or critical limb ischemia, reported an overall CI-AKI incidence of 11.7%. Most recently, Prasad and colleagues[35] performed a meta-analysis on 15 studies, including 11,311 patients undergoing peripheral angiography and intervention. CI-AKI definitions varied in the included studies, and mostly involved either an absolute (>0.5 mg/dL) and/or relative (>25%) change in SCr from baseline. The median contrast volume across the included studies was 138 mL. The rates of reported CI-AKI varied across the 15 studies, ranging from 0% to 45%, with a median of 10.0%. Higher rates of CI-AKI are reported when extensive aortic manipulation is involved, such as in cases of endovascular aneurysm repair (9%–19%).[36]

Structural Interventions

Most structural heart disease interventions have traditionally been performed in patients with advanced age and high comorbidity burden, which make them ineligible or high-risk for surgery. Therefore, CI-AKI (and AKI in general) is a particularly relevant problem in this context. In view of the expanding indications of structural interventions (in particular, transcatheter aortic valve replacement [TAVR]) to intermediate-risk and possibly low-risk patients, the total number of cases of CI-AKI is expected to increase further. This section presents an outline of CI-AKI epidemiology according to the different structural interventions performed in contemporary practice.

Transcatheter aortic valve replacement

Exposure to CM is only one of several factors responsible for AKI in subjects undergoing TAVR for severe aortic stenosis. These include patient comorbidities (age, CKD, diabetes mellitus, peripheral arterial disease, anemia, and so

forth), procedural factors (scraping of atheroma and subsequent atheroembolic showers into the renal arteries secondary to manipulation of large-bore catheters in the aorta), and complications (bleeding, transfusions, hypotension, infections, and so forth). For these reasons, most available literature focuses on TAVR-associated AKI rather than CI-AKI. Contemporary research on TAVR adheres to the Valve Academic Research Consortium 2 (VARC-2) consensus document,[37] which uses an AKIN-based definition and extends the timing for CI-AKI diagnosis up to 7 days postprocedure. Earlier reports, however, utilized heterogeneous definitions of CI-AKI, thus limiting comparisons across them and with current literature.

Trial data. Fig. 4A presents the incidence of AKI across TAVR trials. In PARTNER A,[38] which randomized high-risk patients to TAVR with a balloon-expandable prosthesis or surgical replacement, the 30-day incidence of an increase in SCr to greater than 3 mg/dL was 1.2% and the need for renal replacement therapy was 2.9% in the TAVR arm. These figures were 0% and 1.1%, respectively, in the TAVR arm of the PARTNER B trial,[39] which randomized inoperable patients with aortic stenosis to TAVR or standard therapy. PARTNER 2[40] compared TAVR and surgery in intermediate-risk patients, and observed a 30-day incidence of stage 2 VARC-2/AKIN-defined AKI of 1.3% in the TAVR arm. Finally, PARTNER 3,[41] which focused on low-risk patients, demonstrated a 30-day incidence of stage 2 or 3 VARC-2/AKIN-defined AKI of only 0.4%, and a need for renal replacement therapy of only 0.2% in the TAVR arm.

The U.S. CoreValve Pivotal Trial[42] randomized high-risk patients to TAVR with a self-expandable valve or surgical replacement and observed a 30-day incidence of risk, injury, failure, loss of kidney function, and end-stage kidney disease (RIFLE)-defined AKI (stage was unspecified) of 6.0% in the TAVR group. The SURTAVI trial[43] focused on intermediate-risk patients and reported a 30-day incidence of AKIN-defined CI-AKI stage 2 or stage 3 of 1.7% in the TAVR group. Finally, the Evolut Low Risk Trial[44] reported a 30-day incidence of AKIN-defined CI-AKI stage 2 or 3 of 0.9% in the TAVR arm.

Registry data. The relatively low figures of AKI rates from randomized trials contrast with those reported in real-life TAVR registries (Fig. 4B). The reasons for this discrepancy are multifaceted and stem mainly from the selective reporting of advanced stages of AKI in randomized

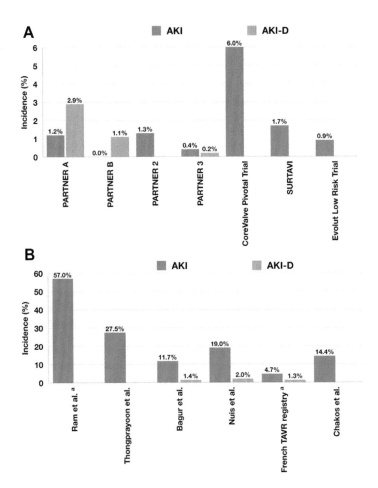

Fig. 4. Incidence of AKI and AKI requiring dialysis (AKI-D) in TAVR (A) trials and (B) registries. [a] Figures reported for the highest-risk groups.

trials and the higher baseline patient risk of AKI in registries. For example, Ram and colleagues[45] report great variability in AKI figures across registries, from 15% to 57%. An analysis from the Mayo Clinic observed an incidence of KDIGO-defined AKI of 27.5% (stage 1: 22.0%; stage 2: 1.6%; and stage 3: 3.9%).[46] Bagur and colleagues[47] conducted a single-center analysis of patients undergoing TAVR with first-generation balloon-expandable prostheses via the transfemoral or transapical approach and observed an incidence of AKI (defined as a reduction of >25% in eGFR within 48 h after TAVR or the need for hemodialysis) of 11.7%, with 1.4% requiring hemodialysis. Nuis and colleagues[48] performed a similar study in patients treated with first-generation self-expandable prostheses and observed an incidence of AKIN-defined AKI of 19%, with 2% requiring renal replacement therapy. A recent meta-analysis on 31 studies, including a total of 13,857 patients, indicated a 30-day incidence of AKI of 14.4%.[49] Finally, a large analysis from the French TAVR registry

(n = 16,969) observed a decrease in the incidence of AKIN-defined AKI (from 4.7% to 3.8%) and need for dialysis (from 1.3% to 0.7%) between the period from 2010 to 2012 and from 2013 to 2015.[50] These findings, which parallel randomized trial data in progressively lower-risk populations, indicate that, as patient comorbidity burden decreases, so does the incidence of post-TAVR AKI.

Mitral interventions
Transcatheter mitral valve interventions are currently represented mainly by percutaneous edge-to-edge repair (MitraClip), a procedure that is contrast-free, so by definition any case of postprocedural AKI is to be linked to noxae different from CM (eg, hypotension or bleeding). There are, however, few data on the incidence of AKI after MitraClip. Taramasso and colleagues[51] reported an incidence of RIFLE-defined AKI stage 2 or 3 of 23.8%, with 6.8% requiring hemodialysis. Spieker and colleagues[52] observed AKIN-defined AKI in 18%;

no patient required renal replacement therapy. On the other hand, CM sometimes is used during transcatheter mitral valve replacement. In a single-center study by Ye and colleagues,[53] AKIN-defined AKI stage 3 requiring hemodialysis was observed in 3.2%. In the largest multicenter registry available to date,[54] AKIN-defined CI-AKI stage 2 or 3 was observed in 6.0% and was higher for valve-in-ring than valve-in-valve (11.1% vs 4.0%; P = .03).

Left atrial appendage closure

Patients undergoing left atrial appendage closure usually present extensive comorbidities (advanced age, CKD, bleeding diathesis, and so forth) that put them at high risk for CI-AKI. In a recent multicenter report by Nombela-Franco and colleagues,[55] median contrast volume was 150 mL. AKIN-defined CI-AKI was observed in 9.0% (7.0% stage 1, 1.1% stage 2, and 0.8% stage 3). Two patients (0.6%) needed renal replacement therapy after the procedure and 1 patient continued during follow-up. Sedaghat and colleagues[56] reported an overall incidence of AKIN-defined CI-AKI of 13.7%, of whom 92.3% were stage 1 and 7.7% were stage 2 or 3. Mean contrast volume in this study was 112 mL ± 90 mL.

IMPLICATIONS

Short-Term Outcomes of Patients with Contrast-Induced Acute Kidney Injury

CI-AKI often is regarded as a transient event, because SCr normalizes within 1 week to 3 weeks in 80% of cases.[57] In a non-negligible proportion, however, CI-AKI is associated with serious adverse outcomes, including progression to kidney failure, need for renal replacement therapy, cardiovascular events, prolongation of hospital stay, and mortality.[58] Weisbord and colleagues[59] reported in-hospital mortality rates of 13.6% and 13.9% for patients who suffered a rise in SCr of greater than or equal to 25% at 24 hours and 48 hours, respectively, after coronary angiography with or without intervention. In the cohort of patients undergoing PCI studied by McCullough and colleagues,[60] the in-hospital mortality rate for patients who developed CI-AKI (increase in SCr >25% within 5 days) was 7.1%, whereas it increased markedly to 35.7% among those who suffered CI-AKI requiring dialysis. Gruberg and colleagues[61] reported an incidence of CI-AKI requiring dialysis of 0.7% in patients undergoing PCI. These patients had an in-hospital mortality of 27.5%, and 23% of those surviving were discharged on a permanent dialysis program. Moreover, Marenzi and colleagues[22] reported

that patients undergoing primary PCI who developed CI-AKI (increase in SCr >0.5 mg/dL) had more complicated clinical course (acute pulmonary edema, need for mechanical ventilation, and major bleeding) and higher mortality (31% vs 0.6%; P<.001). Finally, data from the NCDR CathPCI Registry[17] indicated that the rates of in-hospital death were 0.5%, 9.7%, and 34.3% for patients with no AKIN-defined CI-AKI, CI-AKI, and CI-AKI requiring dialysis, respectively.

Long-Term Outcomes of Patients with Contrast-Induced Acute Kidney Injury

CI-AKI also is associated with a legacy effect on long-term follow-up. McCullough and colleagues[60] reported that the 2-year survival of patients who suffered CI-AKI requiring dialysis after PCI was only 18.8%. Similarly dismal figures were reported by Gruberg and colleagues,[61] who observed a 1-year mortality of 54.5% in subjects who suffered CI-AKI requiring dialysis after PCI. At 1-year follow-up, 75% of the patients who required in-hospital dialysis and were discharged on a permanent dialysis program were still on dialysis. In patients with CKD, even transient renal damage (ie, CI-AKI that subsequently resolves with a return of renal function to baseline) is associated with increased risk for death at 5-year follow-up.[24] In a large cohort from the NCDR CathPCI Registry,[62] AKIN-defined CI-AKI was associated with higher postdischarge risk for death, myocardial infarction, bleeding, recurrent AKI, and AKI requiring dialysis. For each outcome, the highest incidence was within 30 days, although survival curves continued to separate throughout 1-year follow-up.

Economic Implications

As a consequence of the aforementioned observations, the strong association between CI-AKI and increased length of stay and health care costs is not surprising. In the cohort of patients undergoing primary PCI described by Marenzi and colleagues,[22] patients developing CI-AKI had longer hospital stay (13 days ± 7 days vs 8 days ± 3 days; P<.001). Similarly, in the study by Gruberg and colleagues[61] of patients suffering CI-AKI requiring dialysis after PCI, the mean length of stay after intervention was 15.4 days ± 10.3 days, with 7.3 days ± 7.6 days in the intensive care unit, at a cost of $1227/d (the study was published in 2001). Subsequently, Subramanian and colleagues[63] indicated that the average in-hospital cost of CI-AKI was $10,345 and the 1-year cost was $11,812 in 2007. More recent figures (from 2019), derived from a prospective registry of patients undergoing CTO PCI,[64] indicate that patients with CI-AKI can expect a mean length of stay of 6.6 days ± 2.5 days (of which 5.0 days are due to CI-AKI) and a mean cost of $36,244 ± $23,692 (of which $19,357 are attributable to CI-AKI). In such study, CI-AKI represented the third most costly complication, after death and need for cardiac surgery.

SUMMARY

CI-AKI frequently is observed in patients undergoing a variety of catheter-based procedures in interventional cardiology. Although exact estimates and comparisons in the literature have traditionally been hampered by the lack of homogeneous definitions, the recent widespread adoption of validated definitions (AKIN/KDIGO consensus) should facilitate outcome research in the future. CI-AKI is associated with a large burden of morbidity and mortality both in the short term and long term and, therefore, is linked to increased length of stay and health care costs. Accordingly, rapid identification of patients at risk for the development of CI-AKI and control of predisposing factors for this condition is likely to improve clinical outcomes and may help mitigate the increasing costs of health care delivery.

DISCLOSURE

L. Azzalini received honoraria from Abbott Vascular, Guerbet, Terumo, and Sahajanand Medical Technologies; and research support from ACIST Medical Systems, Guerbet, and Terumo. S. Kalra has served as a speaker, consultant, or advisory board member for Boston Scientific, Philips, Abbott Vascular, Abiomed, and Asahi Intecc but has received no honoraria.

REFERENCES

1. Wilhelm-Leen E, Montez-Rath ME, Chertow G. Estimating the risk of radiocontrast-associated nephropathy. J Am Soc Nephrol 2017;28:653–9.
2. McDonald JS, McDonald RJ, Carter RE, et al. Risk of intravenous contrast material-mediated acute kidney injury: a propensity score-matched study stratified by baseline-estimated glomerular filtration rate. Radiology 2014;271:65–73.
3. Azzalini L, Candilio L, McCullough PA, et al. Current risk of contrast-induced acute kidney injury following coronary angiography and intervention: a reappraisal of the literature. Can J Cardiol 2017; 33:1225–8.
4. Azzalini L, Spagnoli V, Ly HQ. Contrast-induced nephropathy: from pathophysiology to preventive strategies. Can J Cardiol 2016;32:247–55.
5. Mehran R, Dangas G, Weisbord SD. Contrast-associated acute kidney injury. N Engl J Med 2019;380: 2146–55.
6. Group AKIW. Kidney Disease: Improving Global Outcomes (KDIGO) - Clinical practice guideline for acute kidney injury. Kidney Int Suppl 2012;2: 1–138.
7. Dharnidharka VR, Kwon C, Stevens G. Serum cystatin C is superior to serum creatinine as a marker of kidney function: a meta-analysis. Am J Kidney Dis 2002;40:221–6.
8. Briguori C, Visconti G, Rivera NV, et al. Cystatin C and contrast-induced acute kidney injury. Circulation 2010;121:2117–22.
9. Quintavalle C, Anselmi CV, De Micco F, et al. Neutrophil gelatinase-associated lipocalin and contrast-induced acute kidney injury. Circ Cardiovasc Interv 2015;8:e002673.
10. Aspelin P, Aubry P, Fransson SG, et al. Nephrotoxic effects in high-risk patients undergoing angiography. N Engl J Med 2003;348:491–9.
11. Sreenivasan J, Zhuo M, Khan MS, et al. Anemia (hemoglobin ≤13 g/dl) as a risk factor for contrast-induced acute kidney injury following coronary angiography. Am J Cardiol 2018;122:961–5.
12. Nijssen EC, Rennenberg RJ, Nelemans PJ, et al. Prophylactic hydration to protect renal function from intravascular iodinated contrast material in patients at high risk of contrast-induced nephropathy (AMACING): a prospective, randomised, phase 3, controlled, open-label, non-inferiority trial. Lancet 2017;6736:1–11.
13. Mehran R, Aymong ED, Nikolsky E, et al. A simple risk score for prediction of contrast-induced nephropathy after percutaneous coronary intervention: development and initial validation. J Am Coll Cardiol 2004;44:1393–9.
14. Azzalini L, Vilca LM, Lombardo F, et al. Incidence of contrast-induced acute kidney injury in a large cohort of all-comers undergoing percutaneous coronary intervention: comparison of five contrast media. Int J Cardiol 2018;273:69–73.
15. Mehta RL, Kellum JA, Shah SV, et al. Acute Kidney Injury Network: report of an initiative to improve outcomes in acute kidney injury. Crit Care 2007; 11:R31.
16. From AM, Al Badarin FJ, McDonald FS, et al. Iodixanol versus low-osmolar contrast media for prevention of contrast induced nephropathy meta-analysis of randomized, controlled trials. Circ Cardiovasc Interv 2010;3:351–8.
17. Tsai TT, Patel UD, Chang TI, et al. Contemporary incidence, predictors, and outcomes of acute kidney injury in patients undergoing percutaneous coronary interventions: insights from the NCDR Cath-PCI registry. JACC Cardiovasc Interv 2014;7:1–9.

18. Inohara T, Kohsaka S, Miyata H, et al. Performance and validation of the U.S. NCDR acute kidney injury prediction model in Japan. J Am Coll Cardiol 2016; 67:1715–22.

19. Gurm HS, Seth M, Dixon SR, et al. Contemporary use of and outcomes associated with ultra-low contrast volume in patients undergoing percutaneous coronary interventions. Catheter Cardiovasc Interv 2019;93:222–30.

20. Slocum NK, Grossman PM, Moscucci M, et al. The changing definition of contrast-induced nephropathy and its clinical implications: insights from the Blue Cross Blue Shield of Michigan Cardiovascular Consortium (BMC2). Am Heart J 2008;163: 829–34.

21. Gurm HS, Seth M, Dixon S, et al. Trends in contrast volume use and incidence of acute kidney injury in patients undergoing percutaneous coronary intervention. JACC Cardiovasc Interv 2018; 11:509–11.

22. Marenzi G, Lauri G, Assanelli E, et al. Contrast-induced nephropathy in patients undergoing primary angioplasty for acute myocardial infarction. J Am Coll Cardiol 2004;44:1780–5.

23. Maioli M, Toso A, Leoncini M, et al. Effects of hydration in contrast-induced acute kidney injury after primary angioplasty: a randomized, controlled trial. Circ Cardiovasc Interv 2011;4:456–62.

24. Maioli M, Toso A, Leoncini M, et al. Persistent renal damage after contrast-induced acute kidney injury: incidence, evolution, risk factors, and prognosis. Circulation 2012;125:3099–107.

25. Kirtane AJ, Doshi D, Leon MB, et al. Treatment of higher-risk patients with an indication for revascularization: evolution within the field of contemporary percutaneous coronary intervention. Circulation 2016;134:422–31.

26. Demir OM, Lombardo F, Poletti E, et al. Contrast-induced nephropathy after percutaneous coronary intervention for chronic total occlusion versus non-occlusive coronary artery disease. Am J Cardiol 2018;122:1837–42.

27. Azzalini L, Ojeda S, Demir OM, et al. Recanalization of chronic total occlusions in patients with vs without chronic kidney disease: the impact of contrast-induced acute kidney injury. Can J Cardiol 2018;34:1275–82.

28. Azzalini L, Poletti E, Lombardo F, et al. Risk of contrast-induced nephropathy in patients undergoing complex percutaneous coronary intervention. Int J Cardiol 2019;290:59–63.

29. Flaherty MP, Pant S, Patel SV, et al. Hemodynamic support with a microaxial percutaneous left ventricular assist device (Impella) protects against acute kidney injury in patients undergoing high-risk percutaneous coronary intervention. Circ Res 2017;120:692–700.

30. Giustino G, Mehran R, Serruys PW, et al. Left main revascularization with PCI or CABG in patients with chronic kidney disease: EXCEL trial. J Am Coll Cardiol 2018;72:754–65.

31. Chalmers N, Jackson RW. Comparison of iodixanol and iohexol in renal impairment. Br J Radiol 1999; 72:701–3.

32. Plaisance BR, Munir K, Share DA, et al. Safety of contemporary percutaneous peripheral arterial interventions in the elderly: insights from the BMC2 PVI (Blue Cross Blue Shield of Michigan Cardiovascular Consortium Peripheral Vascular Intervention) Registry. JACC Cardiovasc Interv 2011;4: 694–701.

33. Arora P, Davari-farid S, Gannon MP, et al. Low levels of high-density lipoproteins are associated with acute kidney injury following revascularization for chronic limb ischemia. Ren Fail 2013;35: 838–44.

34. Kim GS, Ko YG, Shin DH, et al. Elevated serum cystatin C level is an independent predictor of contrast-induced nephropathy and adverse outcomes in patients with peripheral artery disease undergoing endovascular therapy. J Vasc Surg 2012; 61:1223–30.

35. Prasad A, Ortiz-Lopez C, Khan A, et al. Acute kidney injury following peripheral angiography and endovascular therapy: a systematic review of the literature. Catheter Cardiovasc Interv 2016;88: 264–73.

36. Jhaveri KD, Saratzis AN, Wanchoo R, et al. Endovascular aneurysm repair (EVAR)- and transcatheter aortic valve replacement (TAVR)-associated acute kidney injury. Kidney Int 2017;91:1312–23.

37. Kappetein AP, Head SJ, Généreux P, et al. Updated standardized endpoint definitions for transcatheter aortic valve implantation: the Valve Academic Research Consortium-2 consensus document. J Am Coll Cardiol 2012;60:1438–54.

38. Smith CR, Leon MB, Mack MJ, et al. Transcatheter versus surgical aortic-valve replacement in high-risk patients. N Engl J Med 2011;364:2187–98.

39. Leon MB, Smith CR, Mack M, et al. Transcatheter aortic-valve implantation for aortic stenosis in patients who cannot undergo surgery. N Engl J Med 2010;363:1597–607.

40. Leon MB, Smith CR, Mack MJ, et al. Transcatheter or surgical aortic-valve replacement in intermediate-risk patients. N Engl J Med 2016; 374:1609–20.

41. Mack MJ, Leon MB, Thourani VH, et al. Transcatheter aortic-valve replacement with a balloon-expandable valve in low-risk patients. N Engl J Med 2019;380:1695–705.

42. Adams DH, Popma JJ, Reardon MJ, et al. Transcatheter aortic-valve replacement with a self-expanding prosthesis. N Engl J Med 2014;370:1790–8.

43. Reardon MJ, Van Mieghem NM, Popma JJ, et al. Surgical or transcatheter aortic-valve replacement in intermediate-risk patients. N Engl J Med 2017; 376:1321–31.

44. Popma JJ, Deeb GM, Yakubov SJ, et al. Transcatheter aortic-valve replacement with a self-expanding valve in low-risk patients. N Engl J Med 2019;380:1706–15.

45. Ram P, Mezue K, Pressman G, et al. Acute kidney injury post–transcatheter aortic valve replacement. Clin Cardiol 2017;40:1357–62.

46. Thongprayoon C, Cheungpasitporn W, Srivali N, et al. AKI after transcatheter or surgical aortic valve replacement. J Am Soc Nephrol 2016;27: 1854–60.

47. Bagur R, Webb JG, Nietlispach F, et al. Acute kidney injury following transcatheter aortic valve implantation: predictive factors, prognostic value, and comparison with surgical aortic valve replacement. Eur Heart J 2010;31:865–74.

48. Nuis R-JM, Van Mieghem NM, Tzikas A, et al. Frequency, determinants, and prognostic effects of acute kidney injury and red blood cell transfusion in patients undergoing transcatheter aortic valve implantation. Catheter Cardiovasc Interv 2011;77:881–9.

49. Chakos A, Wilson-Smith A, Arora S, et al. Long term outcomes of transcatheter aortic valve implantation (TAVI): a systematic review of 5-year survival and beyond. Ann Thorac Surg 2017;6:432–43.

50. Auffret V, Lefevre T, Van Belle E, et al. Temporal trend in transcatheter aortic valve replacement in France: FRANCE 2 to FRANCE TAVI. J Am Coll Cardiol 2017;70:42–55.

51. Taramasso M, Latib A, Denti P, et al. Acute kidney injury following MitraClip implantation in high risk patients: incidence, predictive factors and prognostic value. Int J Cardiol 2013;169:e24–5.

52. Spieker M, Hellhammer K, Katsianos S, et al. Effect of acute kidney injury after percutaneous mitral valve repair on outcome. Am J Cardiol 2018;122: 316–22.

53. Ye J, Cheung A, Yamashita M, et al. Transcatheter aortic and mitral valve-in-valve implantation for failed surgical bioprosthetic valves: an 8-year single-center experience. JACC Cardiovasc Interv 2015;8:1735–44.

54. Yoon S, Whisenant BK, Bleiziffer S, et al. Transcatheter mitral valve replacement for degenerated bioprosthetic valves and failed annuloplasty rings. J Am Coll Cardiol 2017;70:1121–31.

55. Nombela-Franco L, Rodés-Cabau J, Cruz-Gonzalez I, et al. Incidence, predictors, and prognostic value of acute kidney injury among patients undergoing left atrial appendage closure. JACC Cardiovasc Interv 2018;11:1074–83.

56. Sedaghat A, Vij V, Streit SR, et al. Incidence, predictors, and relevance of acute kidney injury in patients undergoing left atrial appendage closure with Amplatzer occluders: a multicentre observational study. Clin Res Cardiol 2019. [Epub ahead of print].

57. McCullough PA, Sandberg KR. Epidemiology of contrast-induced nephropathy. Rev Cardiovasc Med 2003;4:S3–9.

58. James MT, Samuel SM, Manning MA, et al. Contrast-induced acute kidney injury and risk of adverse clinical outcomes after coronary angiography: a systematic review and meta-analysis. Circ Cardiovasc Interv 2013;6:37–43.

59. Weisbord SD, Kip KE, Saul MI, et al. Defining clinically significant radiocontrast nephropathy. J Am Soc Nephrol 2003;14:280A–1A.

60. McCullough PA, Wolyn R, Rocher LL, et al. Acute renal failure after coronary intervention: incidence, risk factors, and relations to mortality. Am J Med 1997;103:368–75.

61. Gruberg L, Mehran R, Dangas G, et al. Acute renal failure requiring dialysis after percutaneous coronary interventions. Catheter Cardiovasc Interv 2001;52:409–16.

62. Valle JA, Mccoy LA, Maddox TM, et al. Longitudinal risk of adverse events in patients with acute kidney injury after percutaneous coronary intervention: insights from the National Cardiovascular Data Registry. Circ Cardiovasc Interv 2017;10:e004439.

63. Subramanian S, Tumlin J, Bapat B. Economic burden of contrast-induced nephropathy: implications for prevention strategies. J Med Econ 2007; 10:119–34.

64. Salisbury AC, Karmpaliotis D, Grantham JA, et al. In-hospital costs and costs of complications of chronic total occlusion angioplasty. JACC Cardiovasc Interv 2019;12:323–31.

65. Stacul F, van der Molen A, Reimer P, et al. Contrast induced nephropathy: updated ESUR Contrast Media Safety Committee guidelines. Eur Radiol 2011; 21:2527–41.

66. Bellomo R, Ronco C, Kellum JA, et al. Acute renal failure – definition, outcome measures, animal models, fluid therapy and information technology needs: the Second International Consensus Conference of the Acute Dialysis Quality Initiative (ADQI) Group. Crit Care 2004;8:R204–12.

Nonrenal Complications of Contrast Media

Daniel Krause, DO[a], Damien Marycz, MD[b], Khaled M. Ziada, MD[a],*

KEYWORDS

- Contrast media • Anaphylactoid reactions • Chemotoxicity • Preventive treatment

KEY POINTS

- Physiologic reactions to contrast media are related to ionicity and osmolality; these have become less significant with contemporary nonionic iso-osmolar agents.
- Anaphylactoid reactions are caused by release of histamine and other vasoactive substances, but cannot be considered typical or true anaphylactic reactions mediated by IgE antibodies.
- Patients with a previous anaphylactoid reaction to contrast or atopic conditions are at increased risk of adverse reactions and should be targeted for preventive treatment before repeat exposure.
- Although there are few high-quality data on preventive medical therapies for anaphylactoid reactions, observational studies demonstrated the efficacy of a few pharmacologic agents.
- Appropriate preventive treatment to avoid anaphylactoid reactions must include prednisone or methyl prednisolone, with at least 1 dose administered 6 or more hours before contrast exposure.

Injection of contrast media is the foundation of invasive and interventional cardiovascular practice. Iodine-based contrast was first safely used in the 1920s for urologic procedures and examinations. The initially used agents had high ionic and osmolar concentrations, which led to significant side effects, namely, nausea, vomiting, and hypotension. In the 1950s, and with the development of sodium and meglumine salts of tri-iodinated benzoic acid, newer contrast agents had lower ionic concentrations and lower osmolarity. Modifications to the ionic structure and iodine content in the 1980s led to the development of ionic low-osmolar, nonionic low-osmolar, and nonionic iso-osmolar contrast media. By virtue of their nonionic nature and lower osmolality, contemporary contrast agents are better tolerated and produce fewer major side effects in comparison with ionic high-osmolar contrast agents.[1]

Despite the overall safety of iodinated contrast agents, their use may be associated with side effects and complications. Contrast-induced nephropathy is generally a major concern associated with the use of these agents in the cardiac catheterization laboratory and radiology suites (discussed elsewhere in this article). This article is dedicated to the discussion of all nonrenal side effects and complications related to the use of contrast agents.

There are 2 major classes of side effects and complications related to contrast media: physiologic (or chemotoxic) and anaphylactoid reactions. Physiologic or chemotoxic side effects

This article is an update of a version that previously appeared in volume 3, issue 3 (July 2014) of *Interventional Cardiology Clinics*.

[a] Division of Cardiovascular Medicine, Gill Heart & Vascular Institute, University of Kentucky, 900 South Limestone Street, 326 Wethington Building, Lexington, KY 40536-0200, USA; [b] WakeMed Heart and Vascular, 3000 New Beren Avenue, Raleigh, NC 27610, USA

* Corresponding author. Gill Heart & Vascular Institute, 900 South Limestone Street, 326 Wethington Building, Lexington, KY 40536-0200.

E-mail address: khaled.ziada@uky.edu

Twitter: @ziadak (K.M.Z.)

are related to the physical and chemical properties of the agent used, whereas anaphylactoid reactions are probably related to the iodine content (Fig. 1). The various reactions, their clinical presentations, and management strategies are discussed in detail.

PHYSIOLOGIC OR CHEMOTOXIC REACTIONS

Physiologic reactions are related to the chemical properties, volume, and rate of infusion of the contrast agent used. The ionic concentration, osmolality, viscosity, and calcium-binding properties of these contrast agents are responsible for most types of physiologic reactions. Adverse reactions can be classified according to degree of severity into mild, moderate, or severe.[2] Mild reactions to contrast media include nausea, flushing, warmth, and vagal reactions, which may lead to transient and self-limited hypotension. Moderate reactions are of a similar nature, but more protracted and require symptomatic treatment, such as antiemetics and intravenous fluids. A minority of patients complain of chest pain or develop a hypertensive reaction. Severe reactions include more profound hypotension, dysrhythmias, depressed myocardial contractility, seizures, and/or convulsions.

As discussed elsewhere in this article, these reactions were more frequent and more severe with earlier generations of contrast agents, where the agents were ionic and had high osmolality (≤1400 mOsm/kg). Because significant volumes of ionic and osmolar were administered, a sharp increase in serum osmolality ensued, which in turn led to fluid shift from intracellular to the extracellular spaces. Increased intravascular volume led to an in increaser in the left ventricular end-diastolic pressure, pulmonary edema, and cellular dysfunction.[3] Electrophysiologic effects of ionic contrast media included decreased rate of depolarization of the sinoatrial node, PR interval prolongation, and, occasionally, heart block or even ventricular fibrillation. The electrophysiologic effects are likely due to transient hypocalcemia via binding of calcium from the radiopaque anion in addition to calcium-sequestering agents (such as sodium citrate and sodium ethylenediamine tetra-acetic acid) often used in ionic contrast agents of high osmolarity.[4,5] The use of ionic high osmolar contrast agents also resulted in transient depression in myocardial performance and hypotension. This decrease in blood pressure can further lead to myocardial ischemia and circulatory collapse in patients with severe coronary ischemia, decompensated heart failure, or critical aortic stenosis.

ACUTE AND EARLY ANAPHYLACTOID REACTIONS

Anaphylactoid reactions to contrast media are typically divided into 2 classes related to the onset of the reaction in relation to the time of exposure: acute or early reactions occur within 1 hour of delivery, and delayed reactions occur between 1 hour and 7 days after exposure (see Fig. 1).[6]

Manifestations and Incidence

The severity of the acute reactions can range from mild cutaneous reactions (such as rash or urticaria) to severe life-threatening reactions such as circulatory collapse and shock (Table 1).[2] Observational studies in the 1980s showed that mild acute reactions occurred in 3.8% to 12.7% of patients receiving ionic, high-osmolar contrast and in 0.7% to 3.1% of patients receiving nonionic lower osmolar contrast agents. The frequency of immediate severe acute reactions has been reported to be 0.1% to 0.4% for ionic contrast agents and 0.02% to 0.04% for nonionic contrast media.[7–10]

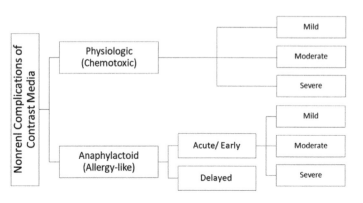

Fig. 1. Types of nonrenal complications of contrast media.

Table 1
Classification of anaphylactoid reactions

Mild	Moderate	Severe
Limited urticaria/itching	Diffuse urticaria/itching	Diffuse edema and/or erythema with hypotension
Limited itchy/scratchy throat	Throat tightness/hoarseness without dyspnea	Laryngeal edema with stridor and/or hypoxia
Mild cutaneous edema	Facial edema, no dyspnea	Facial edema with dyspnea
Sneezing/nasal congestion/ rhinorrhea	Wheezing/bronchospasm without hypoxia	Wheezing/bronchospasm with hypoxia
		Anaphylactic shock (hypotension and tachycardia)

Pathophysiology

The exact pathophysiology causing these reactions is not completely understood and does not seem to result from an observable antigen–antibody interaction. Hence, these reactions are referred to as anaphylactoid, idiosyncratic, allergic-like, or pseudoallergic reactions.[11] Most of these reactions are thought to be related to the release of histamine from basophils and mast cells in addition to other vasoactive substances, or by direct activation of the complement system.[7] In rare cases, IgE antibodies (which are the hallmark of true anaphylaxis) have been reported in the literature as another potential mechanism in the hypersensitivity reactions associated with certain iodinated contrast media.[12,13]

Laboratory Testing

Although not frequently used in clinical practice, the diagnosis can be confirmed at the time of the acute anaphylactoid reaction. Serum levels of histamine may be elevated in some, but not all, individuals after an acute severe anaphylactoid reaction.[14] Tryptase levels may also be elevated in this setting; a blood analysis may be obtained at the time of symptom onset and several days after resolution for comparison.[15]

Skin testing by skin prick, intradermal, and patch methods can be used to identify patients at risk for reactions, particularly those who have reported a prior anaphylactoid reaction and are expected to require subsequent exposure to contrast. Some studies using skin testing have confirmed the cause of acute severe reactions to contrast is immune mediated (and possibly mediated by IgE) and can aid in determining a contrast medium that is less likely to cause a severe reaction in those with a prior history.[16–18] These skin tests should be conducted with caution, because there is some concern

for developing an acute severe allergic reaction to the test itself.

TREATMENT OF ACUTE ANAPHYLACTOID REACTIONS

Although mild reactions are typically transient and self-limited, moderately severe reactions can be more serious, but are usually quick to respond to appropriate therapy. If not recognized and addressed promptly, they may lead to more severe life-threatening reactions. Severe life-threatening reactions to contrast media include facial edema, including of the lips and tongue; laryngeal edema leading to stridor; or severe bronchospasm causing airway compromise, pulmonary edema, arrhythmias, seizures, and circulatory collapse.[19]

It is critically important to distinguish between vasodepressor or vagal reactions and anaphylactoid reactions. Both can result in flushing, nausea, vomiting, and/or hypotension, which can be profound. Vasodepressor reactions differ in that they are associated with bradycardia and heart rate usually less than 50 beats/minutes, whereas hypotension of severe anaphylactoid reactions is commonly associated with tachycardia. The exact cause of vasodepressor reactions to contrast media is not clearly identified, but may be related to chemical properties of the contrast agent on the central nervous system. These reactions may also be related to anxiety associated with the procedure, placing an intravenous access line, or the sight of one's own blood.[20] Distinguishing between vasodepressor and anaphylactoid reactions is crucial, because the treatment options are significantly different.

For mild reactions, patients should be observed after the procedure and discharged only once their symptoms have resolved.

Frequently the symptoms are self-limited, and no additional therapy is needed. In some cases, intravenous ondansetron (4 mg) or prochlorperazine (12.5 mg) can be used to treat persistent nausea and vomiting. Diphenhydramine, 25 to 50 mg intravenously, is often adequate to control pruritus associated with mild rash. Clinical judgment and possibly extended observation are needed to determine whether symptoms will progress and if more aggressive treatment is indicated.

For intermediate reactions, patients require longer and closer observation after the procedure as well as frequent checks on vital signs. In addition to symptomatic treatment of nausea and pruritus, intravenous fluids should be started if there is evidence of hypotension, and intravenous corticosteroids can be considered for diffuse erythema and urticarial reactions.

For severe reactions, it is important to recognize the problem immediately, because these are life-threatening situations. General supportive measures and mobilization of resources (such as calling the intensive care or rapid response nursing teams) are indicated. If intubation is needed, it is usually difficult owing to laryngeal edema and requires expertise.

The initial management of severe acute reactions begins with assessing airway, breathing, and circulation. Oxygen therapy should be started at a rate of 6 to 10 L/min through a rebreathing mask, and intravenous fluids should be administered immediately for hypotension, preferably via a central venous line. Medical therapy should begin with epinephrine, which is the drug of choice for severe allergic reactions to contrast media. Epinephrine increases blood pressure by causing arteriolar and venous vasoconstriction via α-receptor stimulation. It also activates β1 receptors, which causes increases heart rate and myocardial contractility. Epinephrine activation of β2 receptors leads to bronchodilation, which relieves severe bronchospasm. Epinephrine 1:1000 dilution intramuscularly at a dose of 0.1 to 0.3 mL should be given immediately. An autoinjector pen delivers a similar dose and can be effective if that is an available option.[2] If there is severe bronchospasm or airway compromise, a more dilute solution of epinephrine, 1:10,000, can be given at a dose of 1 to 3 mL (0.1–0.3 mg) intravenously, preferably via a central line.[21] In patients with moderate symptomatic bronchospasm without hypotension, an inhaled bronchodilator such as nebulized albuterol can be given. In addition to epinephrine, high-dose intravenous steroids should also be considered at the time of acute severe reactions. The onset of action for steroids is not immediate and can take several hours to be effective, hence the need for epinephrine and volume resuscitation. However, steroids stabilize cell membranes and prevent the biphasic anaphylaxis reaction that can occur from several hours up to 72 hours after acute severe allergic reactions.[22]

Table 2 provides a summary of the main pharmacologic agents, doses and route of administration typically used to treat the main adverse reactions.[2] As discussed elsewhere in this article, to initiate appropriate therapy it is important to distinguish these reactions from vasodepressor responses. Whereas observation and intravascular volume repletion are the common and first steps in both situations, pharmacologic therapy is drastically different. In severe vasodepressor responses, atropine, a competitive inhibitor of acetylcholine, is the drug of choice for reversing bradycardia. Atropine, 1 mg intravenously, should be given immediately, and vital signs should be monitored closely. Repeat administration of atropine maybe needed every 3 to 5 minutes up to a total of 3 mg in adults.[11]

DELAYED REACTIONS

Delayed adverse events occur between 1 hour and 7 days after exposure to contrast media. These delayed reactions are usually mild in comparison with the acute allergic-like reactions and mainly include maculopapular rash, erythema, urticaria, and, rarely, angioedema. Most patients with delayed cutaneous reactions present with macular or maculopapular exanthema. The symmetric drug-related intertriginous and flexural exanthema and drug-related eosinophilia with systemic symptoms are specific exanthemas common to delayed cutaneous reactions to contrast media (Fig. 2).[23]

The incidence of delayed adverse events to contrast media has been reported as up to 14% in some studies.[24] Most of these reactions are thought to be T-cell mediated, and skin biopsies have shown T-cell infiltrate in the dermis.[25,26] Prior immunotherapy for certain malignancies using recombinant IL-2 agents has also been shown to increase the frequency of delayed reactions to iodinated contrast, owing to stimulation of T lymphocytes. One prospective study found that 11.8% of patients receiving IL-2 therapy developed delayed reaction to intravenous contrast, compared with 3.9% in those not receiving IL-2.[27]

A history of allergic reactions also increases the likelihood of a delayed reaction by 2-fold,

Table 2
Commonly used therapeutic agents for the treatment of physiologic and anaphylactoid contrast reactions

Reaction	Medication	Dose	Comments
Nausea	Ondansetron Prochlorperazine	4–8 mg slow IV 2.5–12.5 mg IV	Can cause QT prolongation
Urticaria	Diphenhydramine	25–50 mg oral or IV	Central nervous system depression is common
Bronchospasm (mild)	Albuterol (β2 agonist) Supplemental O$_2$	2 puffs (90 mg/puff) Nasal cannula or face mask	Can repeat in 20 min Common side effects include palpations, tremor, and tachycardia Maintain oximetry >92%
Bronchospasm (moderate or severe)	Epinephrine (1:1000) or epinephrine auto injector (EpiPen) or epinephrine (1:10,000) Albuterol (β2 agonist) Supplemental O$_2$	0.1–0.3 mg (0.1–0.3 mL) IM or 0.3 mg IM (fixed dose) 0.1–0.3 mg (1–3 mL) IV 0.83% nebulized solution, 2.5–5.0 mg once Face mask (6–10 L/min)	Monitor for tachycardia or other arrhythmias Can repeat every few mins, max dose 1 mg Can repeat in 20 min, may cause tachyarrhythmia Monitor pulse oximetry or O$_2$ saturation on blood gases
Laryngeal edema	Epinephrine (1:1000) or epinephrine autoinjector (EpiPen) or epinephrine (1:10,000) Albuterol (β2 agonist) Corticosteroids—methylprednisolone or hydrocortisone	0.1–0.3 mg (0.1–0.3 mL) SC or 0.3 mg IM (fixed dose) 0.1–0.3 mg (1–3 mL) IV 0.83% nebulized solution, 2.5–5.0 mg once 40 mg IV 100–200 mg IV	Monitor for tachycardia or other arrhythmias Can repeat every few mins, max dose 1 mg Can repeat in 20 min, may cause tachyarrhythmia High-dose corticosteroids should generally not be used for >72 h
Symptomatic bradycardia (with or without hypotension)	Atropine	0.5–1 mg IV	Can repeat 0.5–1.0 mg every 3–5 min Maximum dose should not exceed a total of 3 mg

Abbreviations: IM, intramuscularly; IV, intravenously.
Adapted from American College of Radiology Committee on Drugs and Contrast Media. ACR manual on contrast media. Version 10.3. American College of Radiology; 2018. p. 103-109; with permission.

and a previous reaction to contrast medium can increase the risk of late reaction by 1.7- to 3.3-fold.[25] The development of delayed cutaneous reactions may also be related to the contrast agent being used. The use of iso-osmolar contrast agents is associated with a 3 times greater risk of developing a delayed cutaneous reaction than with the use of low osmolar contrast agents.[28] Delayed reactions are usually self-limited and the treatment is based on symptom management, which includes oral antihistamines, emollients, and topical steroids.

Persistent delayed reactions that do not resolve with standard treatment may necessitate further investigation.

It is important to consider delayed reactions to contrast when patients report maculopapular rashes several days after contrast-based procedures. It is not infrequent that the results of the procedure had prompted the initiation of other pharmacologic therapies and that the reactions may be related to the pharmacologic agents rather than the contrast exposure days earlier.

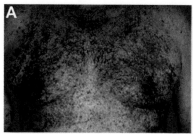
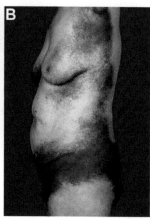

Fig. 2. Typical appearance of maculopapular exanthema (*A*) and symmetric drug-related intertriginous and flexural exanthema (*B*) associated with delayed cutaneous reactions to contrast media. (*From* Brockow K. Immediate and delayed cutaneous reactions to radiocontrast media. Chem Immunol Allergy 2012;97:184; with permission.)

A commonly encountered clinical scenario is patients receiving P2Y12 inhibitors such as clopidogrel after undergoing coronary angiography and stenting. In these settings, and if the reaction is reasonably tolerated, it is prudent to consider a delayed reaction to contrast and continue using the prescribed drugs for a few days, during which the reaction would most commonly subside. If the skin manifestations do not subside within a few days, one must consider the possibility of a reaction to the prescribed drug and instruct the patient to discontinue it while prescribing an alternative.

In difficult clinical situations, skin patch and delayed intradermal testing can also be used to confirm the diagnosis of delayed reactions related to contrast media, with delayed intradermal testing being more sensitive.[7] Because there is high cross-reactivity between different contrast media, patch testing or delayed intradermal testing should also include different contrast media to assess for negative reactions to help identify 1 or more contrast media that can be tolerated with future exposure.

PREVENTION OF CONTRAST REACTIONS
Identifying the Susceptible Patient
Prevention of adverse reactions associated with contrast media begins by recognizing those who are at an increased risk for developing adverse reactions. Although there is no guarantee that a patient is completely immune from developing such reactions, some should be considered high risk, and targeted for preventive measures. The most significant predictor of an adverse reaction to contrast is history of an adverse reaction during a prior exposure. Patients with such history have a 17% to 35% risk of a recurrent reaction with a second contrast

exposure. Patients with atopic conditions, such as asthma and allergic rhinitis, are also at higher risk. Those with asthma have a risk that is approximately 6 times that of the general population. A history of allergic reactions to seafood or shellfish was once thought to be a risk factor for the development of anaphylactoid reactions to iodinated contrast. However, there was no associated increased risk when compared with persons with other food allergies.[29,30] Box 1 summarizes the predisposing risk factors that are commonly considered before contrast exposure.

Pharmacologic Preventive Regimens
Several regimens of premedication have been used to lower the risk of repeat adverse reactions; however, the optimal approach has not been defined. There are no high-quality evidence-based regimens, but the most common premedication regimens are based on corticosteroids and antihistaminic agents. Corticosteroids stabilize the cell membrane through complex signaling mechanisms that result in an increased formation of C1 esterase, ultimately leading to the inhibition of bradykinin, leukotrienes, and other inflammatory mediators responsible for anaphylactoid reactions.[31] Antihistamines reduce pruritus, flushing, and cough by inhibiting the release of proinflammatory cytokines. Whereas the effects of corticosteroids on membrane stabilization can take up to 12 hours to reach peak effect, H_1-blocker antihistamine effects are more rapid, peaking within 30 minutes to 2 hours. Based on several studies,[32,33] the most widely used pretreatment regimen includes the use of oral prednisone, 50 mg at 13 hours, 7 hours, and 1 hour before contrast exposure, along with diphenhydramine, 50 mg, 1 hour before exposure. Meta-analysis of

different steroid regimens supports the use of an alternative regimen: 2 doses of methyl predniso-lone (32 mg) at 6 and 2 hours before contrast injection. The rate of severe reactions in this study was reduced from 0.75% to 0.2% (P = .04).[34] For patients who have had intermediate to severe anaphylactoid reactions to high osmolar ionic contrast, a nonionic low osmolar or preferably a iso-osmolar contrast should be considered for repeat examinations.[35]

Patients with a prior intermediate or severe reaction to contrast media who require emergent contrast-based procedures require special attention and consideration before contrast exposure. To date, no studies have shown that the short-term use of corticosteroids prevent or decrease the risk of anaphylactoid reactions to contrast media. The effects of corticosteroids on circulating mast cells, basophils, and histamine release are primarily seen after 4 to 6 hours based on experimental data.[36–38] When contrast exposure cannot be delayed to allow time for corticosteroids to reach peak effect (eg, with emergency coronary intervention for acute myocardial infarction), some consider only using diphenhydramine, 50 mg intravenously at the time of emergent contrast exposure. It should be noted that the efficacy of H_1 antagonists alone to prevent severe anaphylactoid reactions is not proven, although smaller studies and a subsequent meta-analysis by Delaney and colleagues[39] have challenged that opinion. Fig. 3 illustrates the statistically significant reduction in risk of adverse events with prophylactic antihistamines, although the result seems to be driven by smaller studies.[39]

The recommended premedication regimens for nonemergent and emergent procedures recommended by the American College of Radiology Manual on Contrast Media (version 9, 2013),[40] are summarized in Table 3.

As discussed elsewhere in this article, the evidence underlying the presented regimens for treatment and prevention of serious reactions to contrast media is not of the quality typically required for guideline recommendations. However, it is unlikely that these types of clinical

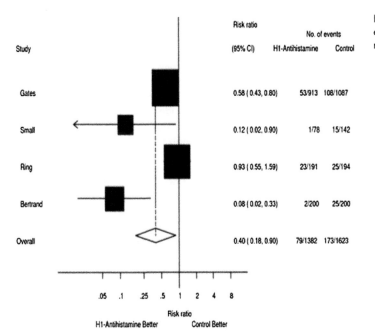

Fig. 3. Meta-analysis demonstrating efficacy of H_1 antagonists in reducing reactions.

Table 3 Pretreatment regimens for patients with prior anaphylactoid contrast reactions	
Elective/Nonurgent Procedures	**Emergent Procedures**
Prednisone, 50 mg PO at 13 h, 7 h, and 1 h before exposure to contrast, *and* diphenhydramine, 50 mg oral, IV or IM 1 h before exposure	*Option 1 - most appropriate* Methylprednisolone, 40 mg or hydrocortisone, 200 mg IV immediately and every 4 h until contrast exposure *and* diphenhydramine, 50 mg IV immediately before exposure
Alternative regimen (for patients unable to receive oral medications) Methylprednisolone, 40 mg IV at 13 h, 7 h, and 1 h before exposure to contrast, *and* diphenhydramine 50 mg IV 1 h before exposure to contrast	*Option 2 - history of allergy to methylprednisolone, aspirin, or NSAIDs, especially if asthmatic* Dexamethasone 7.5 mg IV or betamethasone 6 mg IV immediately and every 4 h until contrast exposure *and* diphenhydramine, 50 mg IV immediately before exposure
	Option 3 - omitting steroids (inadequate time interval for corticosteroid effect) Diphenhydramine, 50 mg IV only, immediately before contrast administration

Abbreviations: IM, intramuscularly; IV, intravenously; NSAID, nonsteroidal anti-inflammatory drug; PO, by mouth.
Data from American College of Radiology Committee on Drugs and Contrast Media. ACR manual on contrast media. 9th edition. Reston (VA): American College of Radiology; 2013. p. 6–11.

problems can be addressed in prospective and randomized placebo-controlled trials. It is possible and probably desirable to explore more innovative approaches regarding timing, dosing and possibly newer classes of medications in carefully designed and actively controlled studies that take into account the potential seriousness of the reactions in a very small fraction of patients.

DISCLOSURE

The authors have no disclosures to report in regard to the content of this article.

REFERENCES

1. McClennan BL. Ionic and nonionic iodinated contrast media: evaluation and strategies for use. AJR Am J Roentgenol 1990;155(2): 225–33.
2. American College of Radiology Committee on Drugs and Contrast Media. ACR manual on contrast media. Version 10.3. American College of Radiology; 2018. p. 103–9.
3. Morcos SK, Thomsen HS. Adverse reactions to iodinated contrast media. Eur Radiol 2001;11:1267–75.
4. Nissen SE, Douglas JS, Dreifus LS, et al. Use of nonionic or low osmolar contrast agents in cardiovascular procedures. J Am Coll Cardiol 1993;21: 269–73.
5. Zuckerman LS, Frichliing TD, Wolf NM, et al. Effect of calcium-binding additives on ventricular fibrillation and repolarization changes during coronary angiography. J Am Coll Cardiol 1987;10:1249–53.
6. Meth MJ, Maibach HI. Current understanding of contrast media reactions and implications for clinical management. Drug Saf 2006;29(2):133–41.
7. Brockow K, Christiansen C, Kanny G, et al. Management of hypersensitivity reactions to iodinated contrast media. Allergy 2005;60:150–8.
8. Katayama H, Yamaguchi K, Kozuka T, et al. Adverse reactions to ionic and nonionic contrast media. A report from the Japanese Committee on the Safety of Contrast Media. Radiology 1990;175:621–8.
9. Wolf GL, Arenson RL, Cross AP. A prospective trial of ionic vs nonionic contrast agents in routine clinical practice: comparison of adverse effects. Am J Roentgenol 1989;152:939–44.
10. Caro JJ, Trindade E, McGregor M. The risks of death and of severe nonfatal reactions with high-vs low-osmolality contrast media: a meta-analysis. Am J Roentgenol 1991;156:825–32.
11. Bush WH, Swanson DP. Acute reactions to intravascular contrast media: types, risk factors, recognition, and specific treatment. AJR Am J Roentgenol 1991;157:1153–61.
12. Mita H, Tadokoro K, Akiyama K. Detection of IgE antibody to a radiocontrast medium. Allergy 1998; 53:1133–40.
13. Kanny G, Maria Y, Mentre B, et al. Case report: recurrent anaphylactic shock to radiographic contrast media. Evidence supporting an exceptional IgE-mediated reaction. Allerg Immunol 1993;25:425–30.

14. Dewachter P, Mouton-Faivre C, Felden F. Allergy and contrast media. Allergy 2001;56:250–1.
15. Laroche D, Vergnaud MC, Sillard B, et al. Biochemical markers of anaphylactoid reactions to drugs. Comparison of plasma histamine and tryptase. Anesthesiology 1991;75:945–9.
16. Trcka J, Schmidt C, Seitz CS, et al. Anaphylaxis to iodinated contrast material: nonallergic hypersensitivity or IgE-mediated allergy? AJR Am J Roentgenol 2008;190:666.
17. Brockow K, Romano A, Aberer W, et al. Skin testing in patients with hypersensitivity reactions to iodinated contrast media—a European multicenter study. Allergy 2009;64:234.
18. Laroche D, Namour F, Lefrancois C, et al. Anaphylactoid and anaphylactic reactions to iodinated contrast material. Allergy 1999;54:13–6.
19. Goss JE, Chambers CE, Heupler FA. Systemic anaphylactoid reactions to iodinated contrast media during cardiac catheterization procedures: guidelines for prevention, diagnosis, and treatment. Cathet Cardiovasc Diagn 1995;34(2):99–104.
20. American College of Radiology Committee on Drugs and Contrast Media. ACR manual on contrast media. 5th edition. Reston (VA): American College of Radiology; 2004. p. 5–77.
21. Cochran ST. Anaphylactoid reactions to radiocontrast media. Curr Allergy Asthma Rep 2005;5:28–31.
22. Tole JW, Lieberman P. Biphasic anaphylaxis: review of incidence, clinical predictors, and observation recommendations. Immunol Allergy Clin North Am 2007;27(2):309–26.
23. Brockow K. Immediate and delayed cutaneous reactions to radiocontrast media. Chem Immunol Allergy 2012;97:180–90.
24. Loh S, Bagheri S, Katzberg RW, et al. Delayed adverse reaction to contrast-enhanced CT: a prospective single-center study comparison to control group without enhancement. Radiology 2010; 255(3):764–71.
25. Bellin MF, Stacul F, Webb JA, et al. Late adverse reactions to intravascular iodine based contrast media: an update. Eur Radiol 2011;21:2305–10.
26. Kanny G, Pichler W, Morisset M, et al. T-cell mediated reactions to iodinated contrast media: evaluation by skin and lymphocyte activations tests. J Allergy Clin Immunol 2005;115:179–85.
27. Choyke PL, Miller DL, Lotze MT, et al. Delayed reactions to contrast media after interleukin-2 immunotherapy. Radiology 1992;183(1):111–4.
28. Sutton AG, Finn P, Grech ED, et al. Early and late reactions after the use of iopamidol 340, ioxaglate 320, and iodixanol 320 in cardiac catheterization. Am Heart J 2001;141(4):677–81.
29. Beary A, Lieberman P, Slavin R. Seafood allergy and radiocontrast media: are physicians propagating a myth? Am J Med 2008;121:158.
30. Lang DM, Alpern MB, Visintainer PF, et al. Increased risk for anaphylactoid reaction from contrast media in patients on beta-adrenergic blockers or with asthma. Ann Intern Med 1991; 115(4):270–6.
31. Lasser EC, Lang JH, Lyon SG, et al. Glucocorticoid-induced elevations of C1-esterase inhibitor: a mechanism for protection against lethal dose range contrast challenge in rabbits. Invest Radiol 1981;16:20–3.
32. Marshall GD Jr, Lieberman PL. Comparison of three pretreatment protocols to prevent anaphylactoid reactions to radiocontrast media. Ann Allergy 1991;67:70.
33. Greenberger PA, Patterson R. The prevention of immediate generalized reactions to radiocontrast media in high-risk patients. J Allergy Clin Immunol 1991;87:867.
34. Lasser EC, Berry CC, Mishkin MM, et al. Pretreatment with corticosteroids to prevent adverse reactions to nonionic contrast media. AJR Am J Roentgenol 1994;162:523–6.
35. Bertrand ME, Esplugas E, Piessens J, et al. Influence of a nonionic, iso-osmolar contrast medium (iodixanol) versus an ionic, low-osmolar contrast medium (ioxaglate) on major adverse cardiac events in patients undergoing percutaneous transluminal coronary angioplasty. Circulation 2000; 101(2):131–6.
36. Saavedra-Delgado AM, Mathews KP, Pan PM, et al. Dose-response studies of the suppression of whole blood histamine and basophil counts by prednisone. J Allergy Clin Immunol 1980;66(6):464–71.
37. Lasser EC. Pretreatment with corticosteroids to prevent reactions to IV contrast: overview and implications. AJR Am J Roentgenol 1988;150:257–9.
38. Miura T, Inagaki N, Yoshida K, et al. Mechanisms for glucocorticoid inhibition of immediate hypersensitivity reactions in rats. Jpn J Pharmacol 1992; 59(1):77–87.
39. Delaney A, Carter A, Fisher M. The prevention of anaphylactoid reactions to iodinated radiological contrast media: a systematic review. BMC Med Imaging 2006. https://doi.org/10.1186/1471-2342-6-2.
40. American College of Radiology Committee on Drugs and Contrast Media. ACR manual on contrast media. 9th edition. Reston (VA): American College of Radiology; 2013. p. 6–11.

Predicting Contrast-Induced Renal Complications

Rachel G. Kroll[1], Prasanthi Yelavarthy, MD[1],
Daniel S. Menees, MD, Nadia R. Sutton, MD, MPH*

KEYWORDS

- Chronic kidney disease • Percutaneous coronary intervention • Contrast-induced nephropathy
- Contrast media • Risk prediction

KEY POINTS

- Identification of patients vulnerable to the development of renal complications is an initial critical step in preventing renal impairment and a new need for dialysis after contrast exposure.
- Contrast media volume, age and sex of the patient, a history of chronic kidney disease and/or diabetes, clinical presentation, and hemodynamic and hydration status are factors known to predict incident contrast-induced nephropathy.
- Many risk models have been created using preprocedural and postprocedural factors to predict the future risk of contrast-induced nephropathy and a new need for dialysis.
- Online calculators can be used to categorize patient risk of contrast-induced nephropathy and a new requirement for dialysis. The online calculator with the highest c-statistic (0.84) for the development of acute kidney injury after contrast-exposure in the setting of percutaneous coronary intervention is the Blue Cross Blue Shield of Michigan Cardiovascular Consortium percutaneous coronary intervention risk calculator for multiple outcomes (bmc2.org/calculators/cin).

INTRODUCTION

Chronic kidney disease (CKD) is a major risk factor for the development of coronary artery disease (CAD), serving as an independent risk factor while also overlapping with other risk factors, such as hypertension and diabetes, which lead to both CKD and CAD.[1] The presence of CAD in patient populations can be asymptomatic or can manifest symptoms ranging from stable angina to acute coronary syndromes (myocardial infarction), cardiogenic shock, and death owing to cardiac arrest.[2] CAD is often diagnosed using noninvasive (computed tomography) or minimally invasive (coronary angiogram) approaches using contrast media (CM). In addition to medical therapy,

percutaneous coronary intervention (PCI) is a minimally invasive approach to restoring myocardial blood flow using angioplasty and coronary artery stenting. Depending on the clinical circumstances, this procedure is used to reduce symptoms owing to coronary artery stenoses or to reduce the risk of future death and myocardial infarction.[3]

PCI, except under rare circumstances, uses intraarterial CM in order to opacify coronary arteries in the cardiac catheterization laboratory.[4] CM, however, can negatively impact renal function, and patients with preexisting CKD are more susceptible to this effect.[5] Once it has been determined that an individual has the potential to benefit from a heart catheterization requiring CM, identifying those at risk for

---

Division of Cardiovascular Medicine, Department of Internal Medicine, University of Michigan, 1500 East Medical Center Drive, SPC 5869, Ann Arbor, MI 48109, USA

[1]These authors contributed equally to this work.
* Corresponding author. Division of Cardiovascular Medicine, University of Michigan Cardiovascular Center, 2A381, SPC 5869, 1500 East Medical Center Drive, Ann Arbor, MI 48109-5869.
E-mail address: nadiaraz@med.umich.edu

Intervent Cardiol Clin 9 (2020) 321–333
https://doi.org/10.1016/j.iccl.2020.02.003

contrast-induced kidney injury is a key initial step in preventing this complication. Systematic clinical application of prediction models for the development of renal complications of PCI raises awareness of an individual patient's risk. Patients at increased risk can receive targeted interventions to reduce the risk of renal complications after PCI, which can potentially be used to monitor the quality and safety of PCI. Because renal complications of PCI are associated with other poor outcome measures, predicting (and subsequently preventing) renal complications of CM exposure is critical to performing PCI safely.

RISK FACTORS FOR CONTRAST-INDUCED ACUTE KIDNEY INJURY
Volume of Contrast Media
The volume of CM administered to patients in a single setting or during multiple administrations within a short duration is strongly associated with the occurrence of contrast-induced nephropathy (CIN) (Fig. 1).[6] CM becomes more concentrated in the hyperosmolar environment of the renal tubules. This increased fluid viscosity reduces renal blood flow, subsequently inducing hypoxia of the renal medulla and cell death because of higher contact time between the cytotoxic CM and endothelial cells.[7]

Risk models have been proposed to predict renal complications of PCI (Table 1) that can be applied in clinical settings, using either calculated creatinine clearance (CCC) or estimated glomerular filtration rate (eGFR). The incidence of CIN has been found to increase when the CM volume/eGFR ratio surpasses 1.[8–10] Similarly, a CM volume (mL) to CCC (mL/min) ratio exceeding 2 is associated with an increased risk of CIN with ratios greater than 3 linked with substantially increased risk.[11–14] Predictive formulas for the maximum safe CM dose have been proposed.[15–17] A recent study by Gurm and colleagues[18] explored using a CM volume less than estimated creatinine clearance to reduce the risk of CIN. This *ultra-low contrast volume* was used in 13% of procedures and was associated with a lower risk of CIN and new-onset dialysis.[18] Other novel strategies of reducing CIN include intravascular ultrasound-guided PCI.[4] CO_2 angiography is not accompanied by renal toxicity but is contraindicated for PCI because of concern for gas embolism, neurotoxicity, and cerebral infarction.[19]

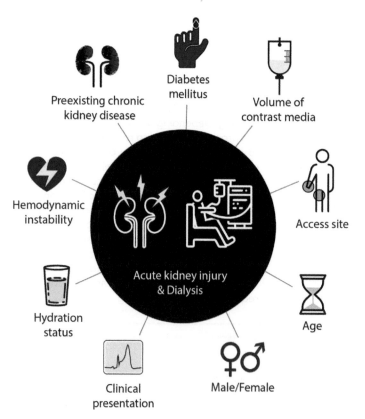

Fig. 1. Risk factors for the development of acute kidney injury and new requirement for dialysis following CM exposure.

Preexisting chronic kidney disease

Diabetes mellitus

Volume of contrast media

Hemodynamic instability

Access site

Hydration status

Age

Acute kidney injury & Dialysis

Clinical presentation

Male/Female

Table 1
Prediction scores for renal complications after percutaneous coronary intervention using preprocedural characteristics

Authors	Population	Outcomes Predicted	Model Variables	Cutoffs	Test Characteristics
Duan et al,[20] 2017	Derivation set 1076 Validation set 701	CIN (≥50% or ≥0.3 mg/dL serum creatinine increase from baseline within 48 h)	Age >75 y, serum creatinine levels, NT-proBNP, hs-CRP, primary PCI	Low risk (0–8) Moderate risk (9–17) High risk (18–26) Very-high risk (≥27)	Prospective observational, single center
Chen et al,[21] 2014	Derivation set 1500 Validation set 1000	CIN (≥25% or ≥0.5 mg/dL serum creatinine increase)	Age ≥70, history of myocardial infarction, diabetes, hypotension, LVEF ≤45%, anemia, eGFR <60, HDL <1 mmol/L, urgent PCI	Low risk (<7) Moderate risk (8–12) High risk (13–16) Very high risk (≥17)	Retrospective, observational, single center in China
Tsai et al,[22] 2014	Derivation set 662,504 Validation set 284,508	CIN (≥50% or ≥0.3 mg/dL 50% serum creatinine increase) and new-onset dialysis	Age, prior 2 wk HF, GFR, diabetes, prior HF/CVD, NSTEMI/UA, STEMI, prior card shock or cardiac arrest, anemia, IABP		Retrospective, observational, multicenter (1253 sites using NCDR Cath/PCI registry)
Ando et al,[23] 2013	481 consecutive patients with STEMI	CIN (≥25% or ≥0.5 mg/dL serum creatinine increase)	AGEF score (adding 1 point to the age/EF [%] ratio if the eGFR was <60 mL/min)		Prospective, observational, single-center study
Gurm et al,[24] 2013	Derivation set 40,001 Validation set 20,572	CIN (≥0.5 mg/dL serum creatinine increase) and new-onset dialysis	PCI indication/status, CAD presentation, cardiogenic shock, heart failure, pre-PCI LVEF, diabetes, age, weight, height, CK-MB, creatinine, hemoglobin, troponin I, and troponin T		Retrospective, observational, multicenter (all nonfederal hospitals in Michigan using BMC2 registry)
Maioli et al,[25] 2010	1218 consecutive patients undergoing PCI (excluding STEMI)	CIN (≥0.5 mg/dL)	Age >73, diabetes, LVEF ≤45%, creatinine ≥1.5 mg/dL or CrCl ≤44 mL/min, posthydration Cr	Low risk (≤3) Moderate risk (4–6) High risk (7–8) Very high risk (≥9)	Prospective, observational, single study in Italy

(continued on next page)

Authors	Population	Outcomes Predicted	Model Variables	Cutoffs	Test Characteristics
Brown et al,[26] 2008	11,141 consecutive patients undergoing PCI	CIN ($\geq$50% or $\geq$2.0 mg/dL serum creatinine increase) or new dialysis	Age $\geq$80, female, diabetes, urgent/emergent, CHF, creatinine, pre-PCI IABP	Risk score 0–37.5	Prospective, observational using the Northern New England Cardiovascular Disease Study Group
Freeman et al,[67] 2002	Derivation set 10,729 Validation set 5863	New-onset dialysis	Peripheral artery disease, diabetes, CKD (Cr >2 mg/dL), heart failure, cardiogenic shock	MRCD = 5 mL × bodyweight (kg)/serum creatinine (mg/dL)	Prospective multicenter using BMC2 registry (8 academic and community hospitals in Michigan)
McCullough et al,[30] 1997	Derivation set 1869 Validation set 1826	New-onset dialysis	CrCl, diabetes, expected contrast dose		Prospective observational, single center

Abbreviations: BMC2, Blue Cross Blue Shield of Michigan Cardiovascular Consortium; BNP, B-type natriuretic peptide; CHF, congestive heart failure; CK-MB, creatine kinase-MB; Cr, creatine; CrCl, creatinine clearance; CRP, C-reactive protein; CVD, cardiovascular disease; HDL, high-density lipoprotein; HF, heart failure; hs, high-sensitivity; IABP, intraaortic balloon pump; LVEF, left ventricular ejection fraction; MRCD, maximum radiographic contrast dose; NCDR, National Cardiovascular Data Repository; NSTEMI, non-ST-elevation myocardial infarction; NT, N-terminal; UA, unstable angina.

Patient Age and Sex

Age is a leading risk factor for the development of renal complications after contrast exposure.[6,20–24] The risk of acute kidney injury (AKI) owing to contrast increases with age, beginning in patients 50 years of age and increasing steadily through age greater than 90.[22] Patients ≥73 years of age are 3 times more likely than younger patients to develop CIN,[25] whereas patients ≥80 years of age have an odds ratio for the development of serious renal dysfunction after contrast exposure of 19.6, relative to patients less than 50 years of age.[26] The AGEF (age, ejection fraction, estimated glomerular filtration rate) score for the prediction of CIN in patients being treated for ST-elevation myocardial infarction (STEMI) includes only 3 clinical variables: age, ejection fraction, and eGFR.[23]

Women have odds of developing renal complications after contrast exposure 1.5 to 2.0 times that of men.[26,27] Furthermore, women without a history of CKD who develop CIN have a higher risk of 1-year mortality.[28] The mechanism underlying the independent association between patient sex or age and renal dysfunction after contrast exposure is unclear and requires further study.

Chronic Kidney Disease

Patients with CKD undergoing PCI carry a higher risk of serious complications of PCI, including mortality.[29–31] Tajti and colleagues[32] described significantly higher rates of in-hospital mortality and major adverse cardiovascular events after PCI in patients with CKD versus those without CKD. Patients with renal dysfunction have a higher risk of requiring repeat urgent revascularization.[33] CKD increases the risk of multiple PCI complications, including development of CIN.

Preexisting CKD is the most significant risk factor in the development of CIN (see Fig. 1).[34–39] Beginning with a baseline eGFR less than 60 mL/min per 1.73 m^2, progressively lower eGFR rates are associated with an increasingly greater risk of CIN.[5,35,40] For example, with an eGFR of 30 mL/min per 1.73 m^2, the risk of developing CIN is as high as 30% to 40%, compared with a risk of 2% for the general population.[39,41]

Diabetes Mellitus

Diabetes often exists concurrently with conditions such as acute coronary syndromes that result in requiring PCI; approximately 1 in 3 patients undergoing PCI have diabetes.[27,40,42] Diabetic patients have a higher risk of developing AKI after PCI, compared with their nondiabetic counterparts.[27,36,43,44] The physiologic mechanisms behind this correlation include increased renal oxygen consumption and reduced medullary oxygenation induced by diabetes combined with reduced renal function triggered by CM.[45] Together, this leads to renal hypoxia, impairing kidney function. Hyperglycemia owing to diabetes may also be an independent predictor of CIN. The incidence of CIN was reported as being significantly higher among diabetic patients with serum glucose ≥150 mg/dL compared with non-hyperglycemic patients.[46]

Clinical Presentation

Myocardial infarction is associated with post-PCI CIN.[47] In several studies, presentation with STEMI was shown to independently predict AKI post-PCI.[22,40] In their analysis of 985,737 patients who underwent PCI, Tsai and colleagues[40] observed a higher incidence of AKI post-PCI in patients who presented with non-STEMI or STEMI when compared with other indications for PCI. Similarly, in their retrospective analysis using the Mayo Clinic PCI registry, Rihal and colleagues[36] reported that acute myocardial infarction within 24 hours before the index PCI, unstable angina, and prior myocardial infarction were all associated with CIN post-PCI. More than half of patients who ultimately experienced CIN initially presented with unstable angina.[36] Impaired left ventricular function (ejection fraction <40%) at the time of PCI is also associated with development of CIN.[23,47–49]

Hemodynamic Instability

Periprocedural hemodynamic instability, indicated by hypotension, requirement for vasopressors, or use of mechanical support devices, is associated with an increased risk of CIN in patients undergoing PCI.[27,47–50] This association between hemodynamic instability and increased risk of CIN is likely multifactorial, related to vasoconstriction and cardiogenic shock resulting in low cardiac output, and the downstream impact on renal perfusion.

Volume Status

CM concentration in the renal medulla correlates with cytotoxicity, and volume expansion with saline has been shown to reduce the risk of subsequent CIN.[51] However, preprocedure hydration status can be challenging to predict based on a physical examination. In addition, emergent procedures using CM in the setting of hypovolemia owing to dehydration or loss of blood volume are sometimes required. Anemia is known to be associated with AKI after PCI in patients with and without preexisting kidney disease.[52] Furthermore, periprocedural bleeding results in anemia, volume depletion, and potentially hemodynamic instability compounding CIN.[53] In these cases, expeditious volume resuscitation and minimization of contrast exposure are important preventive interventions.

Access Site

Recent studies have suggested that a radial access site for coronary intervention and angiography carries a lower risk of bleeding and major vascular complications when compared with using the femoral artery for access.[54–56] In addition, observational and randomized studies have demonstrated that AKI occurs less frequently in patients who undergo invasive procedures with CM via radial arterial access when compared with patients who have their procedure performed via the femoral artery.[57,58] Proposed explanations include that radial access is accompanied by a lower risk of renal atherosclerotic embolization and periprocedural bleeding, which leads to hypovolemia. Radial access has been historically avoided in patients with CKD who may need future dialysis, although practice patterns may be shifting.[56]

Special Populations

The patient population undergoing evaluation for renal transplant that is not yet on dialysis presents unique challenges to health professionals who are faced with determining whether the benefits of PCI outweigh the risks. It is not uncommon in this population for a patient with a glomerular filtration rate (GFR) less than 15 to require PCI because of perceived excessive surgical (renal transplantation) risk without an intervention. A recent study of 535 renal transplant recipients found that a pretransplant PCI was associated with a reduced incidence of adverse posttransplant coronary events, but the association did not reach statistical significance ($P = .06$).[59] In another study, kidney transplant candidates with CKD for whom coronary intervention was recommended but not performed experienced a higher mortality.[60] Other studies have found no difference in mortality between kidney transplant candidates who undergo coronary angiography or PCI and those who do not, suggesting that it may be safer for renal transplant candidates to abstain from these procedures.[61,62] Further studies will be helpful to understand whether the risk of worsening renal function with PCI and potentially expediting a transition to dialysis is outweighed by the benefit of undergoing renal transplantation with a reduced risk of cardiovascular complications.

RENAL COMPLICATIONS OF CONTRAST EXPOSURE

Acute Kidney Injury

The definition of AKI owing to any cause has been defined variably in the literature, ranging from a change in serum creatinine level or change in urine output, to a need for dialysis.[63] Several staging systems have been proposed to provide a consensus definition of AKI, among them the Acute Kidney Injury Network and the Acute Dialysis Quality Initiative (ADQI) systems, both of which use change in serum creatinine or urine output to stratify varied levels of renal failure.[63,64] The ADQI system uses the acronym RIFLE, categorizing patients' renal dysfunction by: patients at risk (R), with injury (I), with failure (F), with sustained loss (L), and with end-stage (E) status in relation to their renal function. When considering CIN specifically, prediction models have used varying definitions of post-PCI AKI, including an increase in serum creatinine of either $\geq 25\%$ or $\geq 50\%$, ≥ 0.5 mg/dL, and ≥ 1.0 mg/dL. Despite these varying definitions, prediction models may be comparable even when CIN definitions differ slightly. Capodanno and colleagues[65] reported that a CM volume to estimated creatinine clearance ratio ≥ 4 reliably predicted the risk of CIN regardless of the definition (either increase in serum creatinine ≥ 0.5 mg/dL or $\geq 25\%$). In the absence of a universal definition of AKI, prediction models can be evaluated through comparison of c-statistics; validated models with a c-statistic of 0.8 or greater could be acceptable for use in practice, if the variables are readily accessible.[66]

New-Onset Dialysis

Development of a need for dialysis because of CIN is correlated with extended duration of hospitalization, long-term renal impairment, and increased short- and long-term mortalities.[26,30,67] Ultimately, reducing the risk of CIN also reduces this more serious complication of newly requiring dialysis, and 5 different risk models have been designed to predict, specifically, the need for dialysis.[22,24,26,30,67] All of these models include preexisting impaired renal function and diabetes as risk factors for requiring dialysis post-PCI. Four of the five models also noted an association between hemodynamic instability and a new need for dialysis post-PCI.[22,24,26,67]

Table 2
Prediction scores for renal complications after percutaneous coronary intervention using postprocedural characteristics

Authors	Population	Outcomes Predicted	Model Variables	Cutoffs	Test Characteristics
Barbieri et al,[72] 2016	2867 consecutive patients undergoing PCI	CIN (≥25% or ≥0.5 mg/dL serum creatinine increase)	Contrast volume/creatinine clearance	V/CrCl ratio ≥6.15 associated with increased risk of CIN	Prospective, observational, single center in Italy
Victor et al,[73] 2014	Derivation set 900 Validation set 300	CIN (≥50% or ≥0.5 mg/dL serum creatinine increase)	GFR, contrast volume, hemoglobin, diabetic microangiopathy, hypotension, albuminuria, peripheral vascular disease		Prospective, observational, single center in India
Tziakas et al,[74] 2013	Derivation set 488 Validation set 200	CIN (≥25% or ≥0.5 mg/dL serum creatinine increase)	CKD, metformin use, prior PCI, peripheral arterial disease, contrast volume ≥300 mL	Low risk (≤2 points) High risk (>2 points)	Prospective, observational, single center in Greece
Chong et al,[75] 2012	770 consecutive patients undergoing PCI	CIN (≥25% or ≥0.5 mg/dL serum creatinine increase)	Age, eGFR, post-PCI CK (for every 500 U/L increase), contrast volume	Low risk (1–3) Moderate risk (4–6) High risk (7–8) Extremely high risk (≥9)	Prospective, observational, single center in Singapore
Tan et al,[76] 2012	1140 consecutive patients undergoing PCI	CIN (≥0.5 mg/dL serum creatinine increase)	Contrast volume/creatinine clearance	V/CrCl ratio >2.62 associated with increased risk of CIN	Prospective, observational, single center in China
Fu et al,[77] 2012	Derivation set 668 Validation set 277	CIN (≥25% or ≥0.5 mg/dL serum creatinine increase)	eGFR, diabetes, LVEF <45%, hypotension, age >70, MI, emergency PCI, anemia, contrast volume >200 mL	Low risk (≤4) Moderate risk (5–8) High risk (9–12) Very high risk (≥13)	Retrospective, observational, single center in China
Ghani & Tohamy,[78] 2009	Derivation set 247 Validation set 100	CIN (≥25% or ≥0.5 mg/dL serum creatinine increase)	Creatinine, shock, female gender, multiple vessel stenting, diabetes	Low (≤4) Moderate (5–8) High (9–12) Very high (≥12)	Prospective, observational, single center in Kuwait

(continued on next page)

Authors	Population	Outcomes Predicted	Model Variables	Cutoffs	Test Characteristics
Mehran et al,[27] 2004	Derivation set 5571 Validation set 2786	CIN (≥25% or ≥0.5 mg/dL serum creatinine increase)	Hypotension, heart failure, CKD, diabetes, age >75 y, anemia, IABP, contrast volume	Low risk ≤5 Moderate risk 6–10 High risk 11–15 Very high risk ≥16	Prospective observational, using Cardiovascular Research Foundation database
Marenzi et al,[47] 2004	208 consecutive AMI patients	CIN (≥0.5 mg/dL serum creatinine increase)	Age >75 y, anterior infarction, time to reperfusion, contrast volume, use of IABP	Risk score 1–5	Prospective observational, single center
Bartholomew et al,[50] 2004	Derivation set 10,481 Validation set 9998	CIN (≥1.0 mg/dL serum creatinine increase)	eGFR <60 mL/min, IABP, urgent/emergent procedure, diabetes, heart failure, hypertension, peripheral artery disease, contrast volume >260 mL	Low risk 0–4 Moderate risk 5–6 High risk 7–8 Very high risk 9–11	Prospective observational, single center

Abbreviations: CK, creatine kinase; V, volume.

Table 3
Online risk calculators

Name	Outcomes	Web Site	Preprocedural or Postprocedural	c-Statistic for AKI	c-Statistic for Dialysis
BMC2 PCI risk calculator	Estimated risk of death, blood transfusion, CIN, and need for new dialysis	https://bmc2.org/calculators/multi	Preprocedural	0.84	0.88
SCAI Risk Assessment Tools (using NCDR PCI registry and Massachusetts Data Analysis Center)	In-hospital mortality, in-hospital bleeding, in-hospital femoral complications, in-hospital AKI, in-hospital dialysis (AKI and dialysis given as an odds ratio vs a healthy 50 year old), 1 y target vessel revascularization, and 30-d readmission	http://www.scai.org/PCIRiskAssessmentTools/default.aspx	Preprocedural (for AKI and need for new dialysis)		
Protected PCI Community AKI calculator using Mehran score[27]	Risk of contrast-induced nephropathy and risk of dialysis	https://www.protectedpci.com/aki-calculator	Preprocedural and postprocedural	0.67	
NCDR AKI and dialysis risk after PCI using Tsai et al[22]	Risk of AKI and risk of dialysis	https://qxmd.com/calculate/calculator_386	Preprocedural	0.71	0.88

Abbreviation: SCAI, Society for Cardiovascular Angiography and Interventions.

PREDICTION TOOLS FOR RISK CALCULATION

Since 1997, nineteen prediction tools have been developed to predict post-PCI renal complications. These risk scores can be divided into 2 groups: those risk scores including preprocedural characteristics (see Table 1) and those including both preprocedural and postprocedural characteristics (Table 2). The risk scores with the preprocedural characteristics can be used as a tool to assess the risk of renal complications before the PCI is performed and to help guide decisions for patients undergoing PCI, especially for those with CKD. The risk scores, including postprocedural characteristics, take into account contrast dose, useful in guiding strategies for contrast volume reduction and potentially for assessing quality. There is considerable overlap in the risk factors that were used to develop these scores.

COMPARISON OF RISK SCORES

In risk models, prediction rules with a c-statistic greater than 0.80 are generally considered acceptable for application in daily practice.[66] The predictive value of the scores in CIN prediction studies varies, with c-statistics between 0.68 and 0.89. Ideally, risk models are validated by the research group in an additional cohort. External validation by another research group is a further step, which could be undertaken before application to clinical practice. Three risk scores have undergone rigorous validation in external cohorts. For example, the risk score by Mehran and colleagues has been validated in 4 studies, with c-statistics ranging between 0.57 and 0.85.[68–70] The score by Bartholomew and colleagues has been validated in 2 additional studies; the predictive score varied between the 2 validation studies.[71] The third risk score that underwent external validation is the score designed by Marenzi and colleagues.[70] Interpretability of these external validation studies, when conflicting, can be limited if the validation studies use a different definition of post-PCI AKI from the original study.

PREDICTION OF ACUTE KIDNEY INJURY AND NEW-ONSET DIALYSIS POSTPERCUTANEOUS CORONARY INTERVENTION

Seventeen of the 19 studies were developed to predict AKI (see Tables 1 and 2). However, the definition of AKI post-PCI varies between studies (increase in serum creatinine $\geq$25%, $\geq$50%, $\geq$0.3 mg/dL, $\geq$0.5 mg/dL, $\geq$1.0 mg/dL, $\geq$2.0 mg/ dL or a combination of 2 of the above) making direct comparisons challenging. There are 5 risk tools that have been developed for the prediction of new-onset dialysis post-PCI. Of these, the risk score by McCullough and colleagues,[30] contains contrast dose and therefore cannot be used preprocedurally. The risk scores by Freeman and colleagues[67] and Gurm and colleagues[24] use baseline patient characteristics, lending the models well to preprocedural prediction of new-onset dialysis post-PCI (Table 3). Using these risk prediction tools to target preventative strategies to high-risk patients systematically provides an opportunity for improved safety and reduced risk of diagnostic angiograms and PCI.

HIGH PERFORMING MODELS

Of the numerous models that are available to predict the risk of contrast-induced nephropathy, the scores by Tsai and colleagues[22] and Gurm and colleagues[24] have the largest derivation and validation sets. Both models use preprocedural characteristics, making it useful to help patients make informed decisions about undergoing a PCI. In addition, they both have online risk calculators (see Table 3), simplifying the process for clinicians to calculate risk. Among the postprocedural risk calculators, the score by Mehran and colleagues[27] is the most widely used; this score is also simple and practical in the clinical setting (see Table 3).

SUMMARY

Prediction of renal complications of contrast exposure is critical to targeting risk-reduction strategies, including hydration, strict contrast volume exposure limits, staging of procedures, and access site choice. Identifying patients vulnerable to this complication using readily available risk-prediction tools is an initial step toward reducing the risk of CIN and a new need for dialysis. A clear understanding of risk factors for CIN also helps identify effective preventive strategies. Prediction of patient subgroups at the highest risk for CIN will determine how to implement impactful interventions to reduce the risk of CIN in the future.

ACKNOWLEDGMENTS

The authors thank Steve Alvey for graphical design.

DISCLOSURE

The authors have no disclosures.

REFERENCES

1. Sarnak MJ, Amann K, Bangalore S, et al. Chronic kidney disease and coronary artery disease: JACC state-of-the-art review. J Am Coll Cardiol 2019;74:1823–38.
2. Libby P, Theroux P. Pathophysiology of coronary artery disease. Circulation 2005;111:3481–8.
3. Levine GN, Bates ER, Blankenship JC, et al. 2011 ACCF/AHA/SCAI guideline for percutaneous coronary intervention: a report of the American College of Cardiology Foundation/American Heart Association Task Force on practice guidelines and the Society for Cardiovascular Angiography and Interventions. Circulation 2011;124:e574–651.
4. Ali ZA, Karimi Galougahi K, Nazif T, et al. Imaging- and physiology-guided percutaneous coronary intervention without contrast administration in advanced renal failure: a feasibility, safety, and outcome study. Eur Heart J 2016;37:3090–5.
5. Mehran R, Nikolsky E. Contrast-induced nephropathy: definition, epidemiology, and patients at risk. Kidney Int Suppl 2006;(100):S11–5.
6. Maioli M, Toso A, Leoncini M, et al. Persistent renal damage after contrast-induced acute kidney injury: incidence, evolution, risk factors, and prognosis. Circulation 2012;125:3099–107.
7. Seeliger E, Sendeski M, Rihal CS, et al. Contrast-induced kidney injury: mechanisms, risk factors, and prevention. Eur Heart J 2012;33:2007–15.
8. Kawatani Y, Kurobe H, Nakamura Y, et al. The ratio of contrast medium volume to estimated glomerular filtration rate as a predictor of contrast-induced nephropathy after endovascular aortic repair. J Med Invest 2018;65:116–21.
9. Nyman U, Bjork J, Aspelin P, et al. Contrast medium dose-to-GFR ratio: a measure of systemic exposure to predict contrast-induced nephropathy after percutaneous coronary intervention. Acta Radiol 2008;49:658–67.
10. Ando G, de Gregorio C, Morabito G, et al. Renal function-adjusted contrast volume redefines the baseline estimation of contrast-induced acute kidney injury risk in patients undergoing primary percutaneous coronary intervention. Circ Cardiovasc Interv 2014;7:465–72.
11. Tan N, Liu Y, Chen JY, et al. Use of the contrast volume or grams of iodine-to-creatinine clearance ratio to predict mortality after percutaneous coronary intervention. Am Heart J 2013;165:600–8.
12. Gurm HS, Dixon SR, Smith DE, et al. Renal function-based contrast dosing to define safe limits of radiographic contrast media in patients undergoing percutaneous coronary interventions. J Am Coll Cardiol 2011;58:907–14.
13. Liu Y, Liu YH, Chen JY, et al. Safe contrast volumes for preventing contrast-induced nephropathy in elderly patients with relatively normal renal function during percutaneous coronary intervention. Medicine (Baltimore) 2015;94:e615.
14. Laskey WK, Jenkins C, Selzer F, et al. Volume-to-creatinine clearance ratio: a pharmacokinetically based risk factor for prediction of early creatinine increase after percutaneous coronary intervention. J Am Coll Cardiol 2007;50:584–90.
15. Cigarroa RG, Lange RA, Williams RH, et al. Dosing of contrast material to prevent contrast nephropathy in patients with renal disease. Am J Med 1989;86:649–52.
16. Brown JR, Robb JF, Block CA, et al. Does safe dosing of iodinated contrast prevent contrast-induced acute kidney injury? Circ Cardiovasc Interv 2010;3:346–50.
17. Marenzi G, Assanelli E, Campodonico J, et al. Contrast volume during primary percutaneous coronary intervention and subsequent contrast-induced nephropathy and mortality. Ann Intern Med 2009;150:170–7.
18. Gurm HS, Seth M, Dixon SR, et al. Contemporary use of and outcomes associated with ultra-low contrast volume in patients undergoing percutaneous coronary interventions. Catheter Cardiovasc Interv 2019;93:222–30.
19. Cho KJ. Carbon dioxide angiography: scientific principles and practice. Vasc Specialist Int 2015;31:67–80.
20. Duan C, Cao Y, Liu Y, et al. A new preprocedure risk score for predicting contrast-induced acute kidney injury. Can J Cardiol 2017;33:714–23.
21. Chen YL, Fu NK, Xu J, et al. A simple preprocedural score for risk of contrast-induced acute kidney injury after percutaneous coronary intervention. Catheter Cardiovasc Interv 2014;83:E8–16.
22. Tsai TT, Patel UD, Chang TI, et al. Validated contemporary risk model of acute kidney injury in patients undergoing percutaneous coronary interventions: insights from the National Cardiovascular Data Registry Cath-PCI Registry. J Am Heart Assoc 2014;3:e001380.
23. Ando G, Morabito G, de Gregorio C, et al. Age, glomerular filtration rate, ejection fraction, and the AGEF score predict contrast-induced nephropathy in patients with acute myocardial infarction undergoing primary percutaneous coronary intervention. Catheter Cardiovasc Interv 2013;82:878–85.
24. Gurm HS, Seth M, Kooiman J, et al. A novel tool for reliable and accurate prediction of renal complications in patients undergoing percutaneous coronary intervention. J Am Coll Cardiol 2013;61:2242–8.
25. Maioli M, Toso A, Gallopin M, et al. Preprocedural score for risk of contrast-induced nephropathy in elective coronary angiography and intervention. J Cardiovasc Med (Hagerstown) 2010;11:444–9.

26. Brown JR, DeVries JT, Piper WD, et al. Serious renal dysfunction after percutaneous coronary interventions can be predicted. Am Heart J 2008;155:260–6.

27. Mehran R, Aymong ED, Nikolsky E, et al. A simple risk score for prediction of contrast-induced nephropathy after percutaneous coronary intervention: development and initial validation. J Am Coll Cardiol 2004;44:1393–9.

28. Iakovou I, Dangas G, Mehran R, et al. Impact of gender on the incidence and outcome of contrast-induced nephropathy after percutaneous coronary intervention. J Invasive Cardiol 2003;15:18–22.

29. Gruberg L, Mehran R, Dangas G, et al. Acute renal failure requiring dialysis after percutaneous coronary interventions. Catheter Cardiovasc Interv 2001;52:409–16.

30. McCullough PA, Wolyn R, Rocher LL, et al. Acute renal failure after coronary intervention: incidence, risk factors, and relationship to mortality. Am J Med 1997;103:368–75.

31. Feng Q, Lu SJ, Klimanskaya I, et al. Hemangioblastic derivatives from human induced pluripotent stem cells exhibit limited expansion and early senescence. Stem Cells 2010;28:704–12.

32. Tajti P, Karatasakis A, Danek BA, et al. In-hospital outcomes of chronic total occlusion percutaneous coronary intervention in patients with chronic kidney disease. J Invasive Cardiol 2018;30:E113–21.

33. Negishi Y, Tanaka A, Ishii H, et al. Contrast-induced nephropathy and long-term clinical outcomes following percutaneous coronary intervention in patients with advanced renal dysfunction (estimated glomerular filtration rate <30 ml/min/1.73 m(2)). Am J Cardiol 2019;123:361–7.

34. McCullough PA, Adam A, Becker CR, et al. Risk prediction of contrast-induced nephropathy. Am J Cardiol 2006;98:27K–36K.

35. McCullough PA. Contrast-induced acute kidney injury. J Am Coll Cardiol 2008;51:1419–28.

36. Rihal CS, Textor SC, Grill DE, et al. Incidence and prognostic importance of acute renal failure after percutaneous coronary intervention. Circulation 2002;105:2259–64.

37. Rich MW, Crecelius CA. Incidence, risk factors, and clinical course of acute renal insufficiency after cardiac catheterization in patients 70 years of age or older. A prospective study. Arch Intern Med 1990; 150:1237–42.

38. Owen RJ, Hiremath S, Myers A, et al. Canadian Association of Radiologists consensus guidelines for the prevention of contrast-induced nephropathy: update 2012. Can Assoc Radiol J 2014;65:96–105.

39. McCullough PA, Sandberg KR. Epidemiology of contrast-induced nephropathy. Rev Cardiovasc Med 2003;4(Suppl 5):S3–9.

40. Tsai TT, Patel UD, Chang TI, et al. Contemporary incidence, predictors, and outcomes of acute kidney injury in patients undergoing percutaneous coronary interventions: insights from the NCDR Cath-PCI registry. JACC Cardiovasc Interv 2014;7:1–9.

41. Gupta RK, Bang TJ. Prevention of contrast-induced nephropathy (CIN) in interventional radiology practice. Semin Intervent Radiol 2010;27:348–59.

42. Gurm HS, Smith D, Share D, et al. Impact of automated contrast injector systems on contrast use and contrast-associated complications in patients undergoing percutaneous coronary interventions. JACC Cardiovasc Interv 2013;6:399–405.

43. Parfrey PS, Griffiths SM, Barrett BJ, et al. Contrast material-induced renal failure in patients with diabetes mellitus, renal insufficiency, or both. A prospective controlled study. N Engl J Med 1989;320:143–9.

44. Weisberg LS, Kurnik PB, Kurnik BR. Risk of radiocontrast nephropathy in patients with and without diabetes mellitus. Kidney Int 1994;45:259–65.

45. Heyman SN, Rosenberger C, Rosen S, et al. Why is diabetes mellitus a risk factor for contrast-induced nephropathy? Biomed Res Int 2013;2013:123589.

46. Turcot DB, Kiernan FJ, McKay RG, et al. Acute hyperglycemia: implications for contrast-induced nephropathy during cardiac catheterization. Diabetes Care 2004;27:620–1.

47. Marenzi G, Lauri G, Assanelli E, et al. Contrast-induced nephropathy in patients undergoing primary angioplasty for acute myocardial infarction. J Am Coll Cardiol 2004;44:1780–5.

48. Dangas G, Iakovou I, Nikolsky E, et al. Contrast-induced nephropathy after percutaneous coronary interventions in relation to chronic kidney disease and hemodynamic variables. Am J Cardiol 2005;95:13–9.

49. Lindsay J, Canos DA, Apple S, et al. Causes of acute renal dysfunction after percutaneous coronary intervention and comparison of late mortality rates with postprocedure rise of creatine kinase-MB versus rise of serum creatinine. Am J Cardiol 2004;94:786–9.

50. Bartholomew BA, Harjai KJ, Dukkipati S, et al. Impact of nephropathy after percutaneous coronary intervention and a method for risk stratification. Am J Cardiol 2004;93:1515–9.

51. Brar SS, Aharonian V, Mansukhani P, et al. Haemodynamic-guided fluid administration for the prevention of contrast-induced acute kidney injury: the POSEIDON randomised controlled trial. Lancet 2014;383:1814–23.

52. Nikolsky E, Mehran R, Lasic Z, et al. Low hematocrit predicts contrast-induced nephropathy after percutaneous coronary interventions. Kidney Int 2005;67:706–13.

53. Ohno Y, Maekawa Y, Miyata H, et al. Impact of periprocedural bleeding on incidence of contrast-induced acute kidney injury in patients treated with percutaneous coronary intervention. J Am Coll Cardiol 2013;62:1260–6.

54. Brener MI, Bush A, Miller JM, et al. Influence of radial versus femoral access site on coronary

angiography and intervention outcomes: a systematic review and meta-analysis. Catheter Cardiovasc Interv 2017;90:1093–104.

55. Rao SV, Hess CN, Barham B, et al. A registry-based randomized trial comparing radial and femoral approaches in women undergoing percutaneous coronary intervention: the SAFE-PCI for Women (Study of Access Site for Enhancement of PCI for Women) trial. JACC Cardiovasc Interv 2014;7:857–67.

56. Sutton NR, Seth M, Lingam N, et al. Radial access use for percutaneous coronary intervention in dialysis patients. Circ Cardiovasc Interv 2020;13(1):e008418.

57. Kooiman J, Seth M, Dixon S, et al. Risk of acute kidney injury after percutaneous coronary interventions using radial versus femoral vascular access: insights from the Blue Cross Blue Shield of Michigan Cardiovascular Consortium. Circ Cardiovasc Interv 2014;7:190–8.

58. Ando G, Cortese B, Russo F, et al. Acute kidney injury after radial or femoral access for invasive acute coronary syndrome management: AKI-MA-TRIX. J Am Coll Cardiol 2017. https://doi.org/10.1016/j.jacc.2017.02.070.

59. De Lima JJ, Gowdak LH, de Paula FJ, et al. Coronary artery disease assessment and intervention in renal transplant patients: analysis from the KiHeart Cohort. Transplantation 2016;100:1580–7.

60. De Lima JJ, Gowdak LH, de Paula FJ, et al. Treatment of coronary artery disease in hemodialysis patients evaluated for transplant-a registry study. Transplantation 2010;89:845–50.

61. Patel RK, Mark PB, Johnston N, et al. Prognostic value of cardiovascular screening in potential renal transplant recipients: a single-center prospective observational study. Am J Transplant 2008;8:1673–83.

62. Jones DG, Taylor AM, Enkiri SA, et al. Extent and severity of coronary disease and mortality in patients with end-stage renal failure evaluated for renal transplantation. Am J Transplant 2009;9:1846–52.

63. Mehta RL, Kellum JA, Shah SV, et al. Acute Kidney Injury Network: report of an initiative to improve outcomes in acute kidney injury. Crit Care 2007;11:R31.

64. Bellomo R, Kellum JA, Ronco C. Defining and classifying acute renal failure: from advocacy to consensus and validation of the RIFLE criteria. Intensive Care Med 2007;33:409–13.

65. Capodanno D, Ministeri M, Cumbo S, et al. Volume-to-creatinine clearance ratio in patients undergoing coronary angiography with or without percutaneous coronary intervention: implications of varying definitions of contrast-induced nephropathy. Catheter Cardiovasc Interv 2014;83:907–12.

66. Ohman EM, Granger CB, Harrington RA, et al. Risk stratification and therapeutic decision making in acute coronary syndromes. JAMA 2000;284:876–8.

67. Freeman RV, O'Donnell M, Share D, et al. Nephropathy requiring dialysis after percutaneous coronary intervention and the critical role of an adjusted contrast dose. Am J Cardiol 2002;90:1068–73.

68. Aykan AC, Gul I, Gokdeniz T, et al. Is coronary artery disease complexity valuable in the prediction of contrast induced nephropathy besides Mehran risk score, in patients with ST elevation myocardial infarction treated with primary percutaneous coronary intervention? Heart Lung Circ 2013;22:836–43.

69. Raposeiras-Roubin S, Abu-Assi E, Ocaranza-Sanchez R, et al. Dosing of iodinated contrast volume: a new simple algorithm to stratify the risk of contrast-induced nephropathy in patients with acute coronary syndrome. Catheter Cardiovasc Interv 2013;82:888–97.

70. Sgura FA, Bertelli L, Monopoli D, et al. Mehran contrast-induced nephropathy risk score predicts short- and long-term clinical outcomes in patients with ST-elevation-myocardial infarction. Circ Cardiovasc Interv 2010;3:491–8.

71. Skelding KA, Best PJ, Bartholomew BA, et al. Validation of a predictive risk score for radiocontrast-induced nephropathy following percutaneous coronary intervention. J Invasive Cardiol 2007;19:229–33.

72. Barbieri L, Verdoia M, Marino P, et al. Contrast volume to creatinine clearance ratio for the prediction of contrast-induced nephropathy in patients undergoing coronary angiography or percutaneous intervention. Eur J Prev Cardiol 2016;23:931–7.

73. Victor SM, Gnanaraj A, Deshmukh R, et al. Risk scoring system to predict contrast induced nephropathy following percutaneous coronary intervention. Indian Heart J 2014;66:517–24.

74. Tziakas D, Chalikias G, Stakos D, et al. Development of an easily applicable risk score model for contrast-induced nephropathy prediction after percutaneous coronary intervention: a novel approach tailored to current practice. Int J Cardiol 2013;163:46–55.

75. Chong E, Shen L, Poh KK, et al. Risk scoring system for prediction of contrast-induced nephropathy in patients with pre-existing renal impairment undergoing percutaneous coronary intervention. Singapore Med J 2012;53:164–9.

76. Tan N, Liu Y, Zhou YL, et al. Contrast medium volume to creatinine clearance ratio: a predictor of contrast-induced nephropathy in the first 72 hours following percutaneous coronary intervention. Catheter Cardiovasc Interv 2012;79:70–5.

77. Fu NK, Yang SC, Chen YL, et al. [Risk factors and scoring system in the prediction of contrast induced nephropathy in patients undergoing percutaneous coronary intervention]. Zhonghua Yi Xue Za Zhi 2012;92:551–4.

78. Ghani AA, Tohamy KY. Risk score for contrast induced nephropathy following percutaneous coronary intervention. Saudi J Kidney Dis Transpl 2009;20:240–5.

Biomarkers of Contrast-Induced Nephropathy:
Which Ones are Clinically Important?

Carmen D'Amore, MD[a], Silvia Nuzzo, PhD[b],
Carlo Briguori, MD, PhD[a],*

KEYWORDS

- Contrast nephropathy • Acute kidney injury • Biomarker • Contrast media

KEY POINTS

- Contrast-induced acute kidney injury (CI-AKI) occurs in 5% to 20% among hospitalized patients.
- Serum creatinine is the gold-standard biomarker to detect CI-AKI, but its delayed kinetic limits its utility as an early biomarker of CI-AKI.
- Novel biomarkers are desirable for an early detection and treatment of CI-AKI in an attempt of improve early and late outcome.

INTRODUCTION

Contrast-induced acute kidney injury (CI-AKI) is an important complication of exposure to iodinated contrast media (CM) used in diagnostic or interventional procedures and may be associated with adverse short- and long-term outcomes.[1,2] CI-AKI is the third most common cause of hospital-acquired AKI after decreased renal perfusion and nephrotoxic medications. The incidence of CI-AKI varies from 5% to 20% among hospitalized patients.[2,3]

CI-AKI is commonly defined as an absolute ($\geq$0.3 or $\geq$0.5 mg/dL) or relative ($\geq$25%) increase of serum creatinine (sCr) compared with baseline values, occurring 48 to 72 hours after the intravascular injection of CM and peaking on the third to the fifth day and returning to baseline within 10 to 14 days.[1] This slow kinetic does not allow an early diagnosis, and it is a potential reason for overlooking CI-AKI and on the contrary, for prolonging hospital stay in most of the patients who will not develop CI-AKI. Furthermore, the increase in sCr depends not only on a reduction of glomerular filtration but

also on the systemic accumulation of sCr generated by skeletal muscles and nonrenal factors (age, sex, muscle mass, and status of hydration),[1] making the increase in sCr values nonspecific for CI-AKI diagnosis. Because of these limitations, other biomarkers have been investigated. In particular, there is a growing interest on biomarkers allowing an earlier and more sensitive detection of kidney damage than sCr. These biomarkers may be classified into 2 groups: (1) those representing changes in renal function (eg, sCr or cystatin C [Cys-C]), and (2) those reflecting structural kidney damage (eg, kidney injury molecule 1, interleukine-18 [IL-18]). Several studies have reported the ability of new urinary/serum biomarkers in the risk stratification, diagnosis, and prediction of prognosis of CI-AKI. A combination of kidney functional and damage biomarkers simultaneously provides an easy method to stratify patients with AKI in 4 groups: (1) no marker change; (2) damage alone; (3) functional change alone, and (4) combined damage and functional changes.[4] Actually, utilization of the new biomarkers of kidney damage has been limited by several reasons:

[a] Interventional Cardiology Unit, Mediterranea Cardiocentro, Via Orazio 2, Naples 80121, Italy; [b] IRCCS, SDN, Via Gianturco 113, Naples 80143, Italy
* Corresponding author. Interventional Cardiology, Clinica Mediterranea, Via Orazio, 2, Naples I-80121, Italy.
E-mail address: carlobriguori@clinicamediterranea.it

Intervent Cardiol Clin 9 (2020) 335–344
https://doi.org/10.1016/j.iccl.2020.02.004
2211-7458/20/© 2020 Elsevier Inc. All rights reserved.

the identification of the best biomarkers for each purpose, uncertainly on the threshold (that may be different in each setting), and limited clinical evidence and costs (**Box 1**).

PATHOPHYSIOLOGY OF CONTRAST-INDUCED ACUTE KIDNEY INJURY

Contrast agents may cause AKI by 2 main mechanisms: (1) direct cellular toxicity and (2) renal hemodynamic effects (**Fig. 1**).[5,6] The cytotoxic effects of CM include apoptosis, a decrease in cell viability, and an increase in brush border and lysosomal enzyme activity; cellular DNA fragmentation; downregulation of signaling molecules involved in cell survival such as Akt and upregulation of signaling molecules in cell death such as the p38 and c-Jun N-terminal kinase members of the mitogen-activated protein kinases and the transcription factor nuclear factor kB as well as caspase activation. Nuclear factor kB and c-Jun N-terminal kinases are believed to be involved in the upregulation of proinflammatory IL-8. An imbalance between vasoconstrictor and vasodilator mediators is implicated in the pathogenesis of CI-AKI. Indeed, the hemodynamics effects are related to an initial increase in renal blood flow, glomerular filtration rate, and urine output, which is directly related to the CM osmolality. Because of increased osmotic load, more sodium is reabsorbed by tubular cells, which itself increases oxygen consumption. Following this transient increase, a decrease (from 10% to 25%) in renal blood flow occurs. The decrease in blood flow seems to be the effect of vasodilators such as adenosine, nitric oxide, atrial natriuretic peptide, and prostaglandine E2. Finally, increased production of reactive oxygen species due to reduced blood flow and increased oxygen consumption

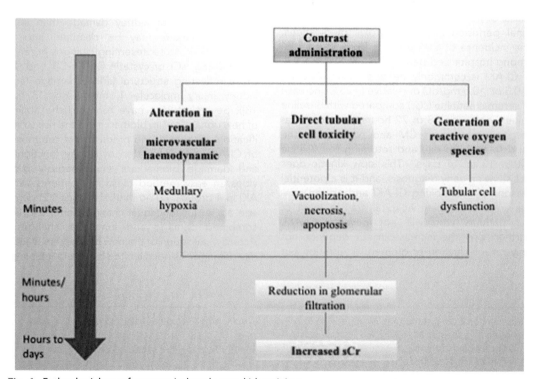

Fig. 1. Pathophysiology of contrast-induced acute kidney injury.

in the medulla are involved in pathogenesis of CI-AKI.

FUNCTIONAL BIOMARKERS

Creatinine

Creatinine is the most widely used endogenous marker of the glomerular filtration rate (GFR), produced at constant rates and freely filtered at the glomerulus, being only 10% to 40% secreted by distal tubule. It is a convenient and cheap marker to measure, but its concentration is affected by several factors, including age, sex, exercise, drugs, muscle mass, nutritional status, and meal intake.[1] Increase of sCr occurs 24 to 72 hours following intravascular CM injection and peaks on the third to the fifth day, returning to baseline within 10 to 14 days. In addition to this slow kinetic, which limits its utility for the early diagnosis of kidney damage, sCr remains within the reference interval until 50% of renal function have been lost.

Microalbuminuria

Microalbuminuria is an important marker of alteration of glomerular structure and function. The term microalbuminuria indicates the urinary albumin in a concentration that is less than the threshold of detection of albumin by conventional urinary dipstick. Its value ranges between 30 and 300 mg/L.[7] Microalbuminuria has been used as a biomarker to investigate attenuation of CI-AKI by N-acetylcysteine.[8] Its limitation, as marker of AKI, is its presence also in chronic renal failure.

Cystatin C

Cys-C is a functional biomarker of glomerular filtration more sensitive to the sCr to detect acute (within 24 hours) changes in renal function. It is a 13 KDa protein, member of the family of cysteine proteinase inhibitors and present in all nucleated cells. Cys-C is filtered by glomeruli and then metabolized in proximal renal tubule cells following megalin-mediated endocytosis.[9] Cys-C is not secreted in the urine by renal tubules. Because of its constant rate of production, its serum concentration is therefore determined by glomerular filtration.[10,11] For these reasons, Cys-C has the potential to be a useful marker in detecting both chronic and acute changes in GFR.[12,13] Furthermore, Cys-C is distributed in the extracellular fluid volume,[14] whereas sCr is distributed in the total body water,[15] which has a 3 times larger volume. Thus, serum Cys-C increases more rapidly than sCr when GFR decreases. The shorted half-life of Cys-C explains the early change in its serum levels compared with sCr.[16] Thus, Cys-C is better than sCr as a marker of GFR.[17]

In CI-AKI, serum Cys-C has been shown to peak as early as 24 hours after CM administration, thereby allowing detection of even small changes in GFR.[18–20]

Briguori and colleagues[21] demonstrated that in 410 patients with chronic kidney disease, undergoing either coronary and/or peripheral angiography and/or angioplasty, a serum Cys-C concentration increase greater than or equal to 10% at 24 hours after CM exposure was associated with a sCr increase greater than or equal to 0.3 mg/dL and was an independent predictor of 1-year major adverse events (MAE), including death and dialysis. Instead, an increase in serum Cys-C less than 10% at 24 hours excluded CI-AKI. This latter finding may allow physicians an earlier discharge of most of the patients, thus avoiding an unnecessary prolonged hospitalization with associated practical and economic advantages.

β_2-Microglobulin

β_2-Microglobulin (β_2M) is an 11.8 kDa protein that is filtered by glomeruli and reabsorbed by the renal proximal tubules.[22] Although low levels of β_2M are found in urine and serum of normal subjects, they increase after renal injury due to decreased reabsorbance by the damaged tubules.

In particular, baseline serum β_2M is a useful predictor of CI-AKI. Nozue and colleagues[23] enrolled 96 patients with stable angina who underwent elective percutaneous coronary intervention (PCI). They measured serum Cys-C and β_2M, and urinary liver-type fatty-acid-binding protein (FABP), β_2M, and N-acetyl-β-D-glucosamide (NAG) before and 1 day after PCI. Patients who experienced CI-AKI (5%) had baseline levels of serum β_2M and Cys-C significantly higher than patients without CI-AKI (4.2 $\pm$ 2.6 vs 2.2 $\pm$ 1.0 mg/L, $P = .0007$ and 1.51 $\pm$ 0.52 vs 1.11 $\pm$ 0.34 mg/L, $P = .013$; respectively). Baseline β_2M>1.26 mg/dL showed a 75% sensitivity and an 80% specificity in predicting CI-AKI. Similar results were reported by Li and colleagues[24] who randomized 424 patients exposed to CM. CI-AKI was defined as an elevation of sCr level by 25% or higher or 0.5 mg/dL greater from baseline within 48 hours. Serum β_2M, Cys-C, and creatinine were measured at 0, 24, and 48 hours of coronary angiography. Before CM exposure, CI-AKI was predicted by both baseline β_2M and CysC. After CM injection CI-AKI was predicted by β_2M, Cys-C, creatinine, and estimated GFR (eGFR). However, multivariate regression analysis confirmed that baseline β_2M and Cys-C were independent predictors for CI-AKI.

Retinol-Binding Protein

Retinol-binding protein (RBP) is a 21 kDa protein that is filtered by glomeruli and is reabsorbed by proximal tubules. It has been shown to be a good marker of AKI; in particular, urinary RBP levels before and after CM injection are used in assessing the efficacy of prevention strategy of AKI with N-acetylcysteine.[25]

STRUCTURAL KIDNEY DAMAGE BIOMARKERS

N-Acetyl-β-D-Glucosamide

NAG is a lysosomal enzyme (>130 kDa) that is produced by the cells of renal proximal tubules. In healthy subjects, NAG is present in small amounts in the urine. The renal tubule disruption leads to its increase in its urine concentration, because of the fact that it is not filtered by glomeruli because of the high weight. However, increased urinary NAG levels may also be the result of increased lysosomal activity without cell disruption.[26]

Ren and colleagues[27] enrolled 590 patients who underwent coronary angiography for both stable and unstable coronary artery disease. Urinary NAG, osmolality, and sCr were sampled before and 1, 2, and 6 days after low-osmolality nonionic CM administration. CI-AKI occurred in 33 patients. In these patients, urinary NAG and sCr levels on days 1 and 2 were significantly higher than at baseline and when compared with patients without CI-AKI. Urinary NAG levels peaked earlier and increased much more than those of sCr in patients with CI-AKI.

Neutrophil Gelatinase–Associated Lipocalin

Neutrophil gelatinase–associated lipocalin (NGAL) is a 25 kDa protein associated with human neutrophil gelatinase that belongs to the superfamily of the lipocalins.[28] The monomeric (mainly) and the heterodimeric forms are the prevalent forms produced by tubules.[29] NGAL is filtered by glomeruli and then reabsorbed by proximal tubules where it is partly degraded by megalin and partly excreted in the urine. The concentration of NGAL in normal subjects is 20 ng/mL, both in serum and in urine. Following renal tubular cell damage, NGAL is released into the plasma and the urine; this causes an increase in its plasma and urine concentration, much early than the increase in sCr concentration.[30] Thus, NGAL has the potential to act as a powerful and independent predictor of AKI.[31–33]

Many clinical studies are reported in the literature concerning the potential role of NGAL as a reliable diagnostic and prognostic biomarker of AKI, because its serum and urinary levels increase earlier and show a better sensitivity than sCr. Some investigators stated the plasma NGAL level to be less specific than its urinary concentration.[34,35]

Recently, Haase and colleagues[35] have demonstrated that, in the absence of the alteration of sCr, patients with increased NGAL had a subclinical AKI and worse prognosis than patients with normal NGAL values. Therefore, NGAL and sCr, probably, reflecting distinct pathophysiological events, could be complementary markers of damage and renal dysfunction. Successively, urinary and serum NGAL (uNGAL and sNGAL) were assessed at 2, 6, 24, and 48 hours after CM exposure in 458 high-risk patients scheduled for coronary or peripheral angiography or angioplasty with an estimated GFR less than or equal to 30 mL/min.[36] Optimal thresholds for CI-AKI (sCr increase $\geq$0.3 mg/dL at 48 hours after CM administration) occurred at 6 hours for both uNGAL ($\geq$20 ng/mL; 97% negative predictive value [NPV]; 27% positive predictive value [PPV]) and sNGAL ($\geq$179 ng/mL; 93% NPV; 20% PPV). Because of the low PPV, high NGAL at 6 hours after CM exposure is a poor predictor of CI-AKI. However, uNGAL less than 20 mg/dL and sNGAL less than 179 mg/dL at 6 hours are reliable markers for ruling out CI-AKI. In addition, Quintavalle and colleagues[37] showed that sNGAL greater than or equal to 179 ng/mL at 6 hours was an independent predictor of 1-year MAE (ie, death, dialysis, nonfatal myocardial infarction, sustained kidney injury, and myocardial revascularization). One-year MAE occurred in 13.5% of patients with sNGAL less than 179 ng/mL and sCr less than 0.3 mg/dL, 29.5% of those with only sNGAL greater than or equal to 179 ng/mL, and 55% of patients with sCr greater than or equal to 0.3 mg/dL. In conclusion, NGAL is a promising marker of AKI, because its increase in the serum and in the urine occurs earlier than the increase of sCr.[34]

Kidney Injury Molecule-1

Kidney injury molecule-1 (KIM-1), a type 1 transmembrane glycoprotein, is recognized as a potential biomarker for detection of ischemic or toxic proximal tubular injury. The extracellular domain of KIM-1 is shed from cell surface by metalloproteinase-dependent process. This shedding with an increased synthesis of KIM-1 is most likely the cause of the increased release of KIM-1 in the urine after AKI.[38,39]

The use of urinary KIM-1 as a biomarker of AKI is based on the fact that there is no KIM-1 expression in the kidney of healthy subjects and on its upregulation in the apical cell membrane of tubule during AKI.[38]

Akdeniz and colleagues[40] enrolled 3200 patients without renal disease that performed coronary angiography. CI-AKI was defined as an increase in serum creatinine by 0.3 mg/dL from a baseline level. The urinary KIM-1 levels were measured before as well as at 6 hours and 48 hours after CM exposure. The authors observed that KIM-1 levels at 6 hours and 48 hours compared with baseline increased significantly in patients with contrast-induced nephropathy but not in control group.

The role of KIM-1 as early CI-AKI biomarker was confirmed also in 145 diabetic patients exposed to CM.[41] In these patients sCr levels were measured before and within 24 and 48 hours after CM injection. Urinary KIM-1 values were assessed at baseline and within 2, 6, 12, 24, and 48 hours after CM exposure. In total, 19 patients developed CI-AKI defined according to the sCr criteria. There was a significant difference between the urinary KIM-1 levels measured 2, 6, 12, 24, and 48 hours after the procedure and those prior the procedure in CI-AKI group. Instead, there was no difference in sCr measured prior and 24 hours after the procedure. Most recently, Wybraniec and colleagues[42] showed that urinary KIM-1 greater than 0.425 ng/mL at 6 hours after CM injection predicted CI-AKI in patients undergoing coronary angiography.

Urinary Interleukin 18

IL-18 is a cytokine doubled in the renal proximal tubules of the kidneys of patients with AKI and is produced from the IL-18 precursor by the action of caspase-1.[43] Urinary levels of IL-18 are increased in acute tubular necrosis but not in prerenal azotemia. It is a sensitive and specific biomarker of AKI.[36] A metanalysis of 23 studies demonstrated that the urine IL-8 is a good biomarker of AKI in patients undergoing cardiac surgery, in patients admitted in intensive care unit and in coronary care unit.[44] As regard as the use of IL-18 as a biomarker of AKI due to CM injection, the studies have conflicting results. He and colleagues[45] enrolled 180 patients scheduled for coronary interventional procedure with a nonionic, low-osmolarity contrast agent. sCr value and eGFR were measured before and within 24 and 48 hours after CM administration. Urine IL-18 levels were measured at baseline and

2, 6, 12, 24, and 48 hours after the coronary interventional procedure. CI-AKI, defined according to sCr criteria, occurred in 8.9% of patients. In the CI-AKI group the IL-18 concentrations were significantly increased from baseline starting from 6 hours after CM injection. On the contrary, sCr levels were not different from baseline to 24 hours, suggesting the potential role of IL-18 for the early CI-AKI detection. The cutoff for the diagnosis of CI-AKI was 815.61 pg/mL (sensitivity and specificity of 87.5% and 62.2%, respectively). Similarly, Ling and colleagues[46] confirmed the role of urinary IL-18 and uNGAL in early diagnosis of CI-AKI and reported that IL-18 was an independent predictor of later MAE. In contrast with these data, BulentGul and colleagues[47] did not find a statistically significant difference in urine IL-18 levels in the 15 cases of patients with CI-AKI compared with patients without CI-AKI; there was no significant difference detected between urinary IL-18 before and after PCI. Finally, in a children population, sNGAL and uNGAL and IL-18 before and after CM administration for radiological examination did not change significantly in 3 consecutive measurements.[48]

Liver-Type Fatty-Acid-Binding Protein

The liver-type fatty-acid-binding protein (L-FABP) is expressed in the proximal tubules of the human kidney and participates in fatty acid metabolism.[49] Two types of FABP are found in the kidney: L-FABP, located in the renal proximal convoluted and straight tubules (it can also be reabsorbed from the glomerular filtrate via megalin, a multiligand proximal tubule endocytic receptor), and heart-type FABP, which is not detected in the urine. Thus, only urinary L-FABP was approved as a tubular injury biomarker. There is a hypoxia responsive element in the promoter region of the L-FABP gene, and other studies reported that urinary L-FABP concentration increased in parallel with decrease in peritubular blood flow, thus L-FABP could detect renal hemodynamic change following administration of CM. Clinical studies have demonstrated that urinary L-FABP at 48 hours after coronary angiography showed a better correlation with the change in eGFR after 1 year to the exposure to CM.[50] Some studies showed that urinary baseline L-FABP levels correlated with occurrence of CI-AKI. Nakamura and colleagues[51] compared urinary L-FABP levels before and after coronary angiography in 66 patients with sCr between 1.2 and 2.5 mg/dL and in 30 healthy volunteers. Before angiography, L-FABP levels were significantly greater

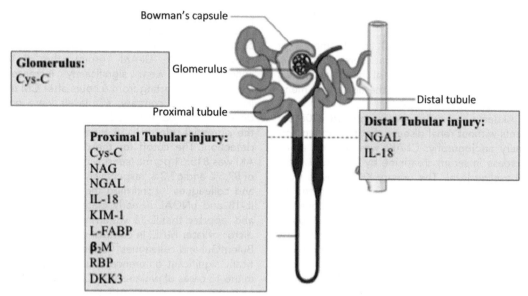

Fig. 2. Production and release of different biomarkers of CI-AKI through the nephron.

in the 13 patients that significantly increased sCr and developed CI-AKI. In particular, Manabe and colleagues[52] found that urinary level greater than or equal to 24.5 µg/g Cr before CM exposure was an independent predictor of CI-AKI (odds ratio 9.10; 95% confidence interval [CI] 3.20–28.9). In addition, measurement of the change in urinary L-FAB before and at 24 hours after cardiac catheterization procedure in patients with mild to moderate renal dysfunction may be an important indicator for risk stratification of onset of cardiovascular events (hazard ratio 4.93; 95% CI 1.27–19.13; P = .021).[53]

Midkine

Midkine (MK) is a 13 KDa growth factor with various biological roles, including inflammation; it regulates cell growth and survival, migration, and antiapoptotic activity in nephrogenesis and development.[54] In the kidney MK is expressed in both proximal tubular cells and distal tubular epithelial cells[55] and to a lesser extent in the endothelial cells[56] and is induced by oxidative stress through the activation of hypoxia-inducible factor 1-alpha.[55] The pathophysiologic roles of MK are diverse, ranging from the occurrence of AKI to progression of chronic kidney disease.[57,58] Malyszko and colleagues[59] investigated whether MK could represent an early biomarker of CI-AKI in 89 patients with normal sCr levels, who underwent percutaneous coronary intervention. Serum MK was evaluated at baseline and after 2, 4, 8, 24, and 48 hours after CM administration; sCR was assessed before

and 24 and 48 hours after CM injection. CI-AKI was defined as an increase in sCr greater than 25% of the baseline 48 hours after PCI and occurred in 10% of the patients. In these patients with CI-KI, a significant increase in serum MK was observed at 2 hours (P<.0019) and 4 hours from the CM exposure; MK return to the baseline value after 24 hours. In this same study, NGAL levels were significantly higher at 2 hours (sNGAL) or 4 hours (uNGAL) after PCI. Cys-C was higher at 8 hours and 24 hours after PCI in patients with CI-AKI.

Dickkopf-3

Dickkopf-3 (DKK3) is a glycoprotein that modulated Wnt/β-catenin signal involved in kidney disease (tubulointerstitial fibrosis) after AKI. In Renal RIP trial,[60] preoperative urinary concentration of DKK3 to creatinine (Dkk3:creatinine) greater than 471 pg/mL was independently associated with significantly higher risk for AKI, persistent renal dysfunction, and dialysis dependency after 90 days. In the same study, the remote ischemic precondition was effective in AKI prevention. Urinary DKK3:creatinine may predict AKI independently to baseline renal function, allowing the identification of patients in whom preventive strategy may be useful.

Miscellany

- Insulin-like growth factor–binding protein 7 and the tissue inhibitor of metalloproteinase-2 are 2 proteins involved in cell cycle arrest that may

Table 1
Potential novel biomarkers of contrast-induced acute kidney injury

Biomarker	Sample	Molecular Weight (kDa)	Site of Lesion	Significant Increase in CI-AKI Patients	Cutoff for CI-AKI Prediction	Method of Detection
Cystatin C	Plasmatic	13	Produced by all nucleated cells, filtered by glomerulus, and reabsorbed by proximal tubule cells	8 h	≥10% increase at 24 h	ELISA and nephelometric and turbidimetric assays
β2Microglobulin	Plasmatic	11.8	Filtered by glomerulus and reabsorbed by the renal proximal tubules	NA	>1.26 mg/dL at baseline	ELISA and nephelometric assays
Retinol-binding protein	Plasmatic	21	Filtered by glomerulus and reabsorbed by the proximal tubule cells	NA	NA	ELISA and nephelometric assays
N-acetyl-β-D-Glucosamide	Urinary	>130	Proximal tubule lysosomal enzyme	24 h	NA	ELISA and spectrophotometric assays
Neutrophil gelatinase-associated lipocalin(NGAL)	Plasma and urinary	25	Expression upregulated in proximal tubule cells after renal injury	2 h	≥20 ng/mL uNGAL ≥179 sNGAL	ELISA, immunoblotting, and turbidimetric assay
Kidney injury molecule-1	Plasma	85	Upregulated in dedifferentiated proximal tubule cells	6 h	>0.425 ng/mL	ELISA and immunoblotting
Interleukin-18	Urinary	18	Expressed in distal tubule cells; expression may be induced in proximal tubules	12 h	(≥25% increase at 24 h)	ELISA
L-fatty acid binding protein	Urinary	14	Expressed in proximal tubule cells	24 h	≥24.5 μg/g	ELISA
Midkine	Serum	13	Expressed in proximal tubule cells	2 h	NA	ELISA
Dickkopf-3	Urinary	na	Tubule cells	Baseline	Dickkopf:creatinine> 471 pg/mL	ELISA

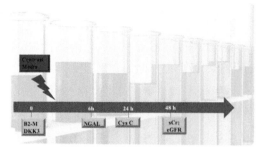

Fig. 3. Timing of clinical detection of the most common biomarkers of CI-AKI. Cys-C, cystatinC; GFR, glomerular filtration rate; NGAL, neutrophil gelatinase–associated lipocalin; sCr, serum creatinine; β2M, β2-microglobulin.

predict AKI. In fact, cell cycle arrest may result as consequence of cellular damage provoked by CM.[54,61] However, there are discordant opinions between the investigators about their use as biomarker to allow their validation.

- Gamma-glutamyl transpeptidase (GGT) is an enzyme on the brush border of the renal proximal tubules, which appear in the urine when damage of the brush border occurs. Increased baseline levels of GGT may predict CI-AKI.[62]

- MicroRNA (miRNA)[63,64] are molecules involved in proliferation, differentiation, and death of cells as well as in the inflammation, suggesting their implication in the pathogenesis of CI-AKI. miRNA molecules have the advantage of their stability in serum, urine, and saliva. For these characteristics and advantages there is more attention about their involvement and ability in CI-AKI prediction.

DISCUSSION

CI-AKI is one of the most frequent causes of renal failure, and it is associated with a prolonged in-hospital stay and an unfavorable outcome. Its incidence will continue to increase due to increasing use in current medicine of iodinate contrast-enhanced percutaneous procedures. sCr is still widely used as a marker of kidney function despite it is a late marker and its concentration may be affected by ages, exercise muscle mass, and some drugs. Hence, there is a need for new early serum and urinary biomarker (Fig. 2, Table 1). Some promising biomarkers have been identified, and they may be able to detect kidney damage before the

expected sCr increase. The most promising marker of CI-AKI are Cys-C, NGAL, KI-1, IL-18, and L-FABP and may give a diagnosis in a subclinical phase of the disease (Fig. 3). However, there are some questions about the accuracy and reliability of these new biomarkers in the context of CIN. In fact, an ideal biomarker should be noninvasive, detectable at early phase of the disease and prognostically relevant, and most important it should be specific for kidney CM injury and have a pathophysiological correlation with the disease. Therefore, to obtain the ideal biomarker may be desirable to carry out multicenter clinical trial to clarify the potential of these biomarkers in different sets of patients.

REFERENCES

1. Tehrani S, Laing C, Yellon DM, et al. Contrast-induced acute kidney injury following PCI. Eur J Clin Invest 2013;43:483–90.
2. McCullough PA, Wolyn R, Rocher LL, et al. Acute renal failure after coronary intervention: incidence, risk factors, and relationship to mortality. Am J Med 1997;103:368–75.
3. Uchino S, Kellum JA, Bellomo R, et al. Acute renal failure in critically ill patients: a multinational, multicentre study. JAMA 2005;294:813–8.
4. McCullough PA, Shaw AD, Haase M, et al. Diagnosis of acute kidney injury using functional and injury biomarkers: workgroup statements from the tenth acute dialysis quality initiative consensus conference. ContribNephrol 2013;182:13–29.
5. Genovesi E, Romanello M, De Caterina R. La nefropatia da mezzo di contrasto in cardiologia. GItalCardiol 2016;17:984–1000.
6. Heyman SN, Rosen S, Rosenberger C. Renal parenchymal hypoxia, hypoxia adaptation, and the pathogenesis of radiocontrast nephropathy. Clin J Am SocNephrol 2008;3:288–96.
7. Ferguson MA, Vaidya VS, Bonventre JV. Biomarkers of nephrotoxic acute kidney injury. Toxicology 2008;245:182–93.
8. Levin A, Pate GE, Shalansky S, et al. N-acetylcysteine reduces urinary albumin excretion following contrast administration: evidence of biological effect. Nephrol Dial Transplant 2007;22:2520–4.
9. Kaseda R, Iino N, Hosojima M, et al. Megalin-mediated endocytosis of cystatin C in proximal tubule cells. BiochemBiophys Res Commun 2007;357:1130–4.
10. Kyhse-Andersen J, Schmidt C, Nordin G, et al. Serum cystatin C, determined by a rapid, automated particle-enhanced turbidimetricmethod, is a better marker than serum creatinine for glomerular filtration rate. ClinChem 1994;40:1921–6.
11. Newman DJ, Thakkar H, Edwards RG, et al. Serum cystatin C measured by automated immunoassay: a

more sensitive marker of changes in GFR than serum creatinine. Kidney Int 1995;47:312–8.

12. Swan SK. The search continues—an ideal marker of GFR. ClinChem 1997;43:913–4.

13. Herget-Rosenthal S, Marggraf G, Hüsing J, et al. Early detection of acute renal failure by serum cystatin C. Kidney Int 2004;66:1115–22.

14. Tenstad O, Roald AB, Grubb A, et al. Renal handling of radiolabelled human cystatin C in the rat. Scand J Clin Lab Invest 1996;56:409–14.

15. Schloerb PR. Total body water distribution of creatinine and urea in nephrectomized dogs. Am J Physiol 1960;199:661–5.

16. Sjostrom P, Tidman M, Jones I. The shorter T1/2 of cystatin C explains the earlier change of its serum level compared to serum creatinine. ClinNephrol 2004;62:241–2.

17. Briguori C, Quintavalle C, Donnarumma E, et al. Novel biomarkers for contrast-induced acute kidney injury. Biomed Res Int 2014;2014:568738.

18. Kuwabara T, Mori K, Mukoyama M, et al. Urinary neutrophil gelatinase-associated lipocalin levels reflect damage to glomeruli, proximal tubules, and distal nephrons. KidneyInt 2009;75: 285–94.

19. Mishra J, Ma Q, Prada A, et al. Identification of neutrophil gelatinase associated lipocalin as a novel early urinary biomarker for ischemic renal injury. J Am SocNephrol 2003;14:2534–43.

20. Mishra J, Mori K, Ma Q, et al. Amelioration of ischemic acute renal injury by neutrophil gelatinase-associated lipocalin. J Am SocNephrol 2004;15:3073–82.

21. Briguori C, Visconti G, Rivera NV, et al. Cystatin C and contrast-induced acute kidney injury. Circulation 2010;121:2117–22.

22. Bernier GM. beta 2-Microglobulin: structure, function and significance. Vox Sang 1980;38:323–7.

23. Nozue T, Michishita I, Mizuguchi I. Predictive value of serum cystatin C, β2-microglobulin, and urinary liver-type fatty acid-binding protein on the development of contrast-induced nephropathy. CardiovascIntervTher 2010;25:85–90.

24. Li S, Zheng Z, Tang X. Preprocedure and postprocedure predictive values of serum β2-microglobulin for contrast-induced nephropathy in patients undergoing coronary computed tomography angiography: a comparison with creatinine-based parameters and cystatin C. J Comput Assist Tomogr 2015;39:969–74.

25. Moore NN1, Lapsley M, Norden AG. Does N-acetylcysteine prevent contrast-induced nephropathy during endovascular AAA repair? A randomized controlled pilot study. J EndovascTher 2006;13: 660–6.

26. de Geus HR, Betjes MG, Bakker J. Biomarkers for the prediction of acute kidney injury: a narrative review on current status and future challenges. ClinKidney J 2012;5:102–8.

27. Ren L, Ji J, Fang Y. Assessment of urinary N-acetyl-β-glucosaminidase as an early marker of contrast-induced nephropathy. J Int Med Res 2011;39: 647–53.

28. Kjeldsen L, Johnsen AH, Sengelov H, et al. Isolation and primary structure of NGAL, a novel protein associated with human neutrophil gelatinase. J BiolChem 1993;268:10425–32.

29. Cai L, Rubin J, Han W, et al. The origin of multiple molecular forms in urine of HNL/NGAL. Clin J Am SocNephrol 2010;5:2229–35.

30. Charlton JR, Portilla D, Okusa MD. A basic science view of acute kidney injury biomarkers. Nephrol Dial Transplant 2014;29:1301–11.

31. Mishra J, Dent C, Tarabishi R, et al. Neutrophil gelatinase-associated lipocalin (NGAL) as a biomarker for acute renal injury after cardiac surgery. Lancet 2005;365:1231–8.

32. Haase M, Bellomo R, Devarajan P, et al, NGAL Meta-analysis Investigator Group. Accuracy of neutrophil gelatinase-associated lipocalin (NGAL) in diagnosis and prognosis in acute kidney injury: a systematic review and meta-analysis. Am J Kidney Dis 2009;54:1012–24.

33. Ronco C. Biomarkers for acute kidney injury: is NGAL ready for clinical use? CritCare 2014;18:680.

34. Clerico A, Galli C, Fortunato A, et al. Neutrophil gelatinase-associated lipocalin (NGAL) as biomarker of acute kidney injury: a review of the laboratory characteristics and clinical evidences. Clin Chem Lab Med 2012;50:1505–17.

35. Haase M, Devarajan P, Haase-Fielitz A, et al. The outcome of neutrophil gelatinase-associated lipocalin-positive subclinical acute kidney injury: a multicenter pooled analysis of prospective studies. J Am CollCardiol 2011;57:1752–61.

36. Parikh CR, Jani A, Melnikov VY, et al. Urinary interleukin-18 is a marker of human acute tubular necrosis. Am J Kidney Dis 2004;43:405–14.

37. Quintavalle C, Anselmi CV, De Micco F, et al. Neutrophil gelatinase-associated lipocalin and contrast-induced acute kidney injury. CircCardiovascInterv 2015;8:e002673.

38. Bonventre JV. Kidney injury molecule-1 (KIM-1): a urinary biomarker and much more. Nephrol Dial Transplant 2009;24:3265–8.

39. Vaidya VS, Ramirez V, Ichimura T, et al. Urinary kidney injurymolecule-1: a sensitive quantitative biomarker for early detection of kidney tubular injury. Am J Physiol Renal Physiol 2006;290:F517–29.

40. Akdeniz D, Celik HT, Kazanci F. Is kidney injury molecule 1 a valuable tool for the early diagnosis of contrast-induced nephropathy? J Investig Med 2015;63:930–4.

41. Li W, Yu Y, He H, et al. Urinary Kidney injury molecule-1 as an early indicator to predict contrast induced acute Kidney injury in patients with diabetes mellitus undergoing percutaneous coronary intervention. Biomed Rep 2015;3:509–12.

42. Wybraniec MT, Chudek J, Bożentowicz-Wikarek M. Prediction of contrast-induced acute kidney injury by early post-procedural analysis of urinary biomarkers and intra-renal Doppler flow indices in patients undergoing coronary angiography. J IntervCardiol 2017;30:465–72.

43. Melnikov VY, Ecder T, Fantuzzi G, et al. Impaired IL-18 processing protects caspase-1-deficient mice from ischemic acute renal failure. J Clin Invest 2001;107:1145–52.

44. Liu Y, Guo W, Zhang J, et al. Urinary interleukin 18 for detection of acute kidney injury: a meta-analysis. Am J Kidney Dis 2013;62:1058–67.

45. He H, Li W, Qian W, et al. Urinary interleukin-18 as an early indicator to predict contrast-induced nephropathy in patients undergoing percutaneous coronary intervention. ExpTher Med 2014;8:1263–6.

46. Ling W, Zhaohui N, Ben H, et al. Urinary IL-18 and NGAL as early predictive biomarkers in contrast-induced nephropathy after coronary angiography. NephronClinPract 2008;108:c176–81.

47. BulentGul CB, Gullulu M, Oral B, et al. Urinary IL-18: a marker of contrast-induced nephropathy following percutaneous coronary intervention? ClinBiochem 2008;41:544–7.

48. Lichosik M, Jung A, Jobs K. Interleukin 18 and neutrophil-gelatinase associated lipocalin in assessment of the risk of contrast-induced nephropathy in children. Cent Eur J Immunol 2015;40:447–53.

49. Veerkamp JH, Peeters RA, Maatman RG. Structural and functional features of different types of cytoplasmic fatty acid-binding proteins. BiochimBiophysActa 1991;1081:1–24.

50. Fujita D, Takahashi M, Doi K. Response of urinary liver-type fatty acid-binding protein to contrast media administration has a potential to predict one-year renal outcome in patients with ischemic heart disease. Heart Vessels 2015;30:296–303.

51. Nakamura T, Sugaya T, Node K. Urinary excretion of liver-type fatty acid-binding protein in contrast medium-induced nephropathy. Am J Kidney Dis 2006;47:439–44.

52. Manabe K, Kamihata H, Motohiro M. Urinary liver-type fatty acid-binding protein level as a predictive biomarker of contrast-induced acute kidney injury. Eur J Clin Invest 2012;42:557–63.

53. Kamijo-Ikemori A, Hashimoto N, Sugaya T. Elevation of urinary liver-type fatty acid binding protein after cardiac catheterization related to cardiovascular events. Int J NephrolRenovasc Dis 2015;8:91–9.

54. Brew K, Nagase H. The tissue inhibitors of metalloproteinases (TIMPs): an ancient family with structural and functional diversity. BiochimBiophysActa 2010;1803:55–71.

55. Sato W, Kadomatsu K, Yuzawa Y, et al. Midkine is involved in neutrophil infiltration into the tubulointerstitium in ischemic renal injury. J Immunol 2001;167:3463–9.

56. Kosugi T, Yuzawa Y, Sato W, et al. Midkine is involved in tubulointerstitial inflammation associated with diabetic nephropathy. Lab Invest 2007;87:903–13.

57. Kato K, Kosugi T, Sato W, et al. Growth factor Midkine is involved in the pathogenesis of renal injury induced by protein overload containing endotoxin. ClinExpNephrol 2011;15:346–54.

58. Okubo S, Niimura F, Matsusaka T, et al. Angiotensinogen gene null-mutant mice lack homeostatic regulation of glomerular filtration and tubular reabsorption. KidneyInt 1998;53:617–25.

59. Malyszko J, Bachorzewska-Gajewska H, Koc-Zorawska E. Midkine: a novel and early biomarker of contrast-induced acute kidney injury in patients undergoing percutaneous coronary interventions. Biomed Res Int 2015;2015:879509.

60. Schunk SJ, Zarbock A, Meersch M, et al. Association between urinary dickkopf-3, acute kidney injury,and subsequent loss of kidneyfunction in patients undergoing cardiac surgery: an observational cohort study. Lancet 2019;394:488–96.

61. Kashani K, Al-Khafaji A, Ardiles T, et al. Discovery and validation of cell cycle arrest biomarkers in human acute kidney injury. CritCare 2013;17:R25.

62. Oksuz F, Yarlioglues M, Cay S, et al. Predictive value of gamma-glutamyltransferase levels for contrast-induced nephropathy in patients with ST-segment elevation myocardial infarction who underwent primary percutaneous coronary intervention. Am J Cardiol 2015;116:711–6.

63. Weber JA, Baxter DH, Zhang S, et al. The microRNA spectrum in 12 body fluids. ClinChem 2010;56:1733–41.

64. Aguado-Fraile E, Ramos E, Conde E, et al. A pilot study identifying a set of microRNAs as precise diagnostic biomarkers of acute kidney injury. PLoS One 2015;10:e0127175.

Implications of Renal Disease in Patients Undergoing Peripheral Arterial Interventions

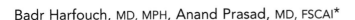

Badr Harfouch, MD, MPH, Anand Prasad, MD, FSCAI*

KEYWORDS

- Claudication • Critical limb ischemia • Peripheral arterial disease
- Peripheral arterial intervention • Chronic renal disease

KEY POINTS

- Peripheral arterial disease (PAD) is common among patients with renal impairment and tends to have a subclinical course with progression.
- Chronic kidney disease (CKD) not only is an independent risk factor of PAD but also an important predictor of poor limb and cardiovascular outcomes and mortality compared to patients with no CKD.
- Despite its lower sensitivity in CKD patients, the ankle-brachial index (ABI) remains the test of choice to assess for PAD. Further tests, such as toe-brachial index and exercise ABI, are reasonable in specific subgroups.
- Invasive angiography is an essential tool to localize disease and guide endovascular therapy. CKD patients have increased risk of developing contrast-induced acute kidney injury; however, effective preventive parameters have been established.
- Prevention and early diagnosis of PAD are decisive steps in CKD patients to improve outcomes and decrease mortality.

DEFINITIONS

Peripheral arterial disease (PAD) is a progressive disorder, characterized by stenosis and/or occlusion of arteries other than those that supply the heart (coronary artery disease).[1,2] Although other disease processes can lead to narrowing of the limb arteries (eg, inflammation and thrombosis) as well as symptoms of arterial insufficiency, atherosclerosis is by far the most prevalent etiology. This is implied in the American Heart Association (AHA) definition of PAD as an atherosclerotic disease that affects the arteries supplying the legs.[3] These definitions apply to patients with renal disease, who represent an important and growing population. Despite that some degree of renal impairment may exist even in patients with glomerular filtration rate (GFR) greater than 60 mL/min, most of the reported studies in this article defined chronic kidney disease (CKD) as GFR less than 60 mL/min for more than 6 months and stratified patients further based on the dependence on dialysis.

EPIDEMIOLOGY AND TRENDS

According to the Centers for Disease Control and Prevention, approximately 8.5 million people in the United States have PAD, including 12% to 20% of individuals older than age 60.[4] PAD is prevalent in patients with CKD,

Division of Cardiology, Department of Medicine, UT Health San Antonio, MC 7872, 8300 Floyd Curl Drive, San Antonio, TX 78229-3900, USA
* Corresponding author.
E-mail address: Prasada@uthscsa.edu

Intervent Cardiol Clin 9 (2020) 345–356
https://doi.org/10.1016/j.iccl.2020.02.007
2211-7458/20/Published by Elsevier Inc.

particularly among those with end-stage renal disease (ESRD) requiring dialysis. At the same time, renal impairment appears common in the presence of PAD.[5] PAD and CKD have unique association and it has been demonstrated that CKD is an independent risk factor for PAD.[6] CKD remains underappreciated, however, as a risk factor for PAD in contemporary guidelines.[7]

Among adults over 40 years old with estimated GFR less than 60 mL/min, the National Health and Nutrition Examination Survey data report a PAD prevalence of 24%.[8] The Chronic Renal Insufficiency Cohort Study data show a PAD prevalence of 7% among CKD nondialysis adult patients and 17% to 48% in dialysis patients.[9] Higher rates of PAD among CKD patients are attributed to greater penetrance of traditional risk factors, such as diabetes, hypertension, dyslipidemia, advanced age, and smoking and renal-specific factors as well.

Dialysis duration, low dialysis adequacy (Kt/V), hypoalbuminemia, low parathyroid hormone, hyperphosphatemia, inflammation, and malnutrition were identified by a cross-sectional analysis of the US Renal Data System as kidney-specific risk factors of PAD.[10] Patients with microalbuminuria and reduced GFR were found to have increased prevalence of PAD compared with those with reduced GFR alone.[11]

The increased reported cases of PAD among CKD patients in the literature also might be explained by the increased screening. The 2005 Kidney Disease Outcomes Quality Initiative guidelines recommend screening (including physical examination with assessment of arterial pulse and skin integrity) at the time of dialysis initiation.[6]

PATHOPHYSIOLOGY

The typical characteristics of PAD in patients with CKD include diffuse calcified atherosclerosis. Implicated mechanisms include increased inflammation with oxidative stress, impaired angiogenesis, and uremic vasculopathy associated with CKD.[12] Severely calcified lesions, in particular, represent a challenge for revascularization, and calcification is a predictor of restenosis postintervention. This pathologic finding is seen in up to a third of CKD patients and is nearly ubiquitous in those with ESRD.[13] Vascular calcification is characteristic of aging but is accelerated in CKD and in diabetes mellitus. Although localized intimal calcification is a feature of atherosclerosis, extensive, widely disseminated medial calcification, often visible on plain radiograph imaging, is a common presenting feature of lower extremity PAD[14] (Fig. 1).

Vascular calcification is a common complication in patients with uremia, due in part to disturbed mineral metabolism and the therapies used to control it but also due to a complex,

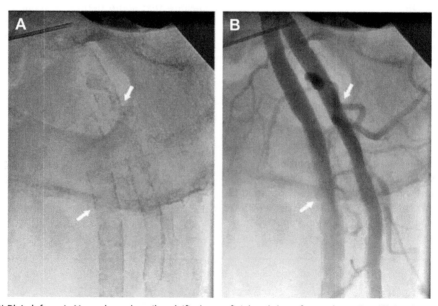

Fig. 1. (A) Plain left groin X-ray shows heavily calcified superficial and deep femoral arteries. (B) Angiography of the same vessels shows no high-grade lesion despite the severe calcification. In both panels left arrow points to the superficial femoral artery, right arrow points to the deep femoral artery.

active process of osteogenesis in vascular smooth muscle cells. Cardiovascular calcifications in patients with CKD are more prevalent, progressive, extensive, and severe compared with those in the non-CKD population.

There are in general 2 types of vascular calcification:

1. Atherosclerotic plaque occurs within the intimal layer. Calcification of the lesions is common but exhibits a patchy, discontinuous course along the artery. Arterial intimal calcification (AIC) is advanced atherosclerosis, driven by cellular necrosis, inflammation, and lipid deposition (Fig. 2).
ESRD-specific risks for AIC include elevated serum phosphate, lower serum albumin, higher calcium intake, and hemodialysis duration. These are the same factors listed previously as kidney-specific risk factors for PAD.
2. Mönckeberg sclerosis occurs in the medial wall (or tunica media). Calcification increases vascular stiffness and reduces vascular compliance. Arterial medial calcification is observed in elastic lamella of the medial layer of conduit arteries.[15]
Calcification, in particular AIC, poses challenges for both surgical and endovascular therapy. Endovascular

treatment strategies often are ineffective due to challenges in vessel expansion after angioplasty, risks of perforation, and need for adjuvant atherectomy. Atherectomy to modify or remove plaque has been the mainstay approach to vessel preparation or in some cases definitive therapy in calcified lesions (Fig. 3 shows an example of atherectomy in a CKD patient). A prominent risk of atherectomy remains distal embolization and the associated consequences of tissue bed ischemia. Novel technologies to address vascular calcification, including delivery of lithotripsy to the vessel wall to fracture calcium, seem promising.[14,16]

CLINICAL PRESENTATION

The symptoms and signs of PAD are variable, and usually they are the same nature in patients with and without renal impairment; however, the initial presenting symptoms differ significantly between CKD and non-CKD patients.

Patients with PAD may be asymptomatic, may experience the classic symptom of claudication, or may present with advanced disease, including critical limb ischemia (CLI). Previous studies have demonstrated that a majority of patients with confirmed PAD do not have

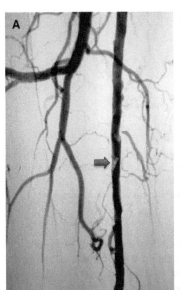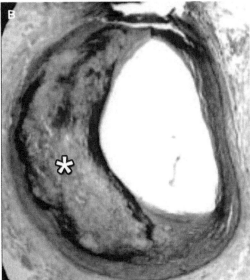

Fig. 2. (A) Angiography of the femoral artery shows diffuse patchy calcified lesion. (B) Arterial cross-sectional microscopic view shows severe intimal calcification. The arrow in (A) points to a patchy calcified lesion in the superior femoral artery. The asterisk in (B) marks the severe arterial intima calcification.

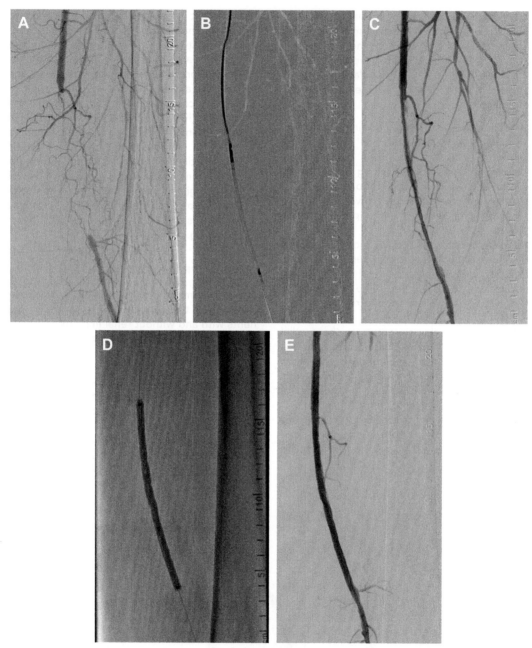

Fig. 3. (A) Chronic total occlusion in the left superficial femoral artery in a CKD patient who presented with CLI. (B: pre-atherectomy, C: post-atherectomy) Lesion crossed using Medtronic (Dublin, Ireland) Viance crossing catheter followed by successful directional atherectomy. (D) Paclitaxel-coated balloon (6 mm × 120 mm) angioplasty was applied to the long lesion. (E) Postintervention angiography shows successful revascularization.

typical claudication but have other non–joint-related limb symptoms (atypical leg symptoms) or are asymptomatic.[7] Conversely, CKD patients are more likely to present with threatening ischemia due to more diffuse and distal disease compared with those who have normal renal function, possibly reflecting the high prevalence of coexistent diabetes in this population. Using the femoral vessels for dialysis access is relatively rare and is considered a last choice due to the high risk of complications. Usually, creating a dialysis access in the lower extremity may worsen or reveal a subclinical PAD in intermittent hemodialysis patients.[17]

DIAGNOSTIC STUDIES

Regardless of the presence of renal disease, the ankle-brachial index (ABI) is widely considered the standard diagnostic tool for PAD, with values less than 0.9 generally considered a diagnostic value. Greater prevalence of calcified vessels in CKD patients raises concerns regarding the utility of this test in these patients due to increased vessel stiffness and increased pressures. In this context, consideration of alternate tests, such as toe-brachial index (TBI) and pulse volume recording, may be appropriate.[6]

Exercise treadmill ABI testing is important to objectively measure functional limitations attributable to leg symptoms and is useful in establishing the diagnosis of lower extremity PAD in the symptomatic patient when resting ABIs are normal (1–1.4) or borderline (0.91–0.99). TBI less than 0.7 is used to establish diagnosis of PAD in the setting of noncompressible arteries (ABI 1.40) and also may be used to assess perfusion in patients with suspected CLI.[7]

DIAGNOSTIC IMAGING AND INVASIVE STUDIES

There are no randomized controlled trials or guidelines regarding invasive testing and/or revascularization for CKD patients with PAD, specifically, who are diagnosed and managed similarly to the general PAD population but with some considerations. Acute limb ischemia in CKD patients is managed emergently by anticoagulation and revascularization procedure (endovascular or surgical) if the limb is salvageable or by amputation if the injury is irreversible. Further testing (beyond ABI, exercise ABI, and TBI) is reserved only for PAD patients who have intermittent claudication and have failed optimal guideline-directed medical therapy (GDMT) as well as progressive ambulation.[7]

Ideally, tests and procedures should be minimized for all patients in general, more importantly for CKD patients, especially those not on dialysis, to avoid exposure to additional nephrotoxic material. This applies specifically to anatomic evaluation by angiography, which provides an opportunity to intervene over other diagnostic imaging studies, unless a surgical procedure is planned.

REVASCULARIZATION

The presence of heavily calcified lesions makes endovascular therapy challenging. Crossing the lesion with a guide wire or a device and achieving enough dilatation can be difficult because of severe calcification.[18] As discussed previously, vessel recoil, dissection, and perforation all are increased in the presence of calcified lesions. Bypass surgery in patients with CKD also may pose challenges, including poor distal targets and need for concomitant endarterectomy. In cases of long occlusions or heavy calcium, bypass surgery has been the preferred approach.[19] Advances in endovascular technology and techniques, however, continue to expand the patient subsets that can be treated with peripheral endovascular intervention (PVI). An endovascular procedure is a reasonable first line in patients with CLI and there are data to support this approach in patients with CKD.[7,20–22]

PVI for PAD management has been increasing among CKD patients compared with surgical revascularization. In a large review (2002–2012) on the national trend of in hospital outcome post-revascularization in hemodialysis patients, there were 77,049 endovascular procedures and 29,556 surgical procedures. Endovascular procedures increased by nearly 3-fold, whereas there was a reciprocal decrease in surgical revascularization. Post-procedure complication rates were relatively stable in persons undergoing endovascular procedures but nearly doubled in those undergoing surgery. Unfortunately, no short-term mortality improvement was seen post–endovascular procedures.[23]

No randomized studies evaluating percutaneous versus surgical revascularization techniques have been conducted in CKD patients with PAD. Most of the available studies concluded that percutaneous methods are preferred in CKD patients, but outcomes are worse among patients with higher rates of repeated percutaneous angioplasty, subsequent surgical revascularization, or limb loss and death. In a retrospective analysis, dialysis patients who underwent percutaneous compared with surgical revascularization experienced higher limb salvage rates. Perioperative morbidity and mortality were higher among CKD patients undergoing surgical procedures.[6] CKD patients with PAD are considered high risk patients in general and they were more likely to be managed conservatively compared with the PAD patient with no CKD. O'Hare and colleagues[24] showed in a study that patients with CLI and GFR less than 60 mL/min were less likely to undergo a revascularization procedure compared with those with better kidney function and instead were more likely to be managed medically or undergo amputation. Nevertheless, for all groups, including those with CKD, patients who underwent revascularization experienced lower mortality rates than the other groups.

An endovascular approach also was found preferable in CKD patients and in dialysis patients, more specifically, as a first-choice therapeutic option. In a prospective study, 42 patients (18 of them were dialysis patients) with superficial femoral artery lesions were treated successfully by primary stent placement. The primary patency, primary assisted patency, limb salvage, and survival rates of the dialysis group were similar to those of the nondialysis group.[21]

PVI generally was considered the most favorable treatment option for ESRD with CLI. In a comparative analysis for in-hospital outcomes in ESRD, patients treated for CLI compared with subjects with normal renal function; 774 patients were studied. The first-line treatment strategies in ESRD patients (102) were PVI in 64%, bypass surgery in 13%, patch plasty in 11%, and no vascular intervention in 13%. In non-ESRD (672) patients, PVI was applied in 48%, bypass surgery in 27%, patch plasty in 13%, and no vascular intervention in 11%. ESRD noticeably increased the risk of in hospital death (odds ratio [OR] 2.62; 95% CI, 1.19–5.79; P [0.017]) and amputation (OR 3.14; 95% CI, 1.35–7.31; P [0.008]).[22]

Despite more complex anatomy, ESRD patients who were treated with PVI as initial therapy did not have significant restenosis rate compared with nondialysis patients. In a prospective study in Japan, 226 patients (118 dialysis patients) had endovascular approach as the first therapeutic option. Dialysis was a predictive factor of amputation and all-cause mortality, not restenosis, however.[25]

Endovascular therapy was found a reasonable first-line treatment option for renal transplant patients as well. In a retrospective study (2003–2010) to assess endovascular therapies in kidney transplant patients with CLI, 28 patients underwent 57 angioplasties. Limb salvage and 1-year survival rates were 83% and 82%, respectively. No measurable change in transplant kidney function was seen, despite higher repeat interventions.[26]

ACUTE KIDNEY INJURY POST–PERIPHERAL VASCULAR ANGIOGRAPHY AND ANGIOPLASTY: ETIOLOGY AND PREVENTION

The incidence of acute kidney injury (AKI) post-PVI in patients presenting with CLI is increasing in general, particularly in CKD and heart failure patients, and was found independently associated with increased in hospital mortality.[27] There are 3 known major causes of AKI post–peripheral vascular angiography (PVA) and/or Post-PVI, including renal atheroemboli, renal hypoperfusion due to hemodynamic instability, and contrast-induced AKI (CI-AKI). The first 2 causes may be relatively rare, and the main management is supportive when they occur. CI-AKI is the most common etiology and is the only potentially preventable factor. CKD patients have an increased risk of developing CI-AKI, which may persist and on rare occasions triggers dialysis dependence temporarily or permanently.[28]

CI-AKI incidence and preventive measures have been well described in patients undergoing coronary angiography; however, the incidence of CI-AKI post-PVA/PVI is poorly described in the literature. In a large systematic review, the median incidence of CI-AKI post-PVA/PVI was 10% with significant variation based on the patients' risk factors.[29]

CI-AKI preventive measures post-PVA/PVI are the same ones applied in the setting of coronary angiography or intervention and are based on maintaining adequate periprocedural hydration, avoiding nephrotoxic agents (such as nonsteroidal anti-inflammatory drugs and metformin for 24–48 hours), minimizing contrast volume, and using less nephrotoxic contrast media, such as low-osmolal or preferably iso-osmolal contrast agents. In patients with CLI, use of antibiotics also may be an important cause of renal dysfunction.

Despite the absence of randomized controlled trials that have directly evaluated the role of fluids versus placebo in the prevention of AKI, intravenous (IV) fluids expansion has been considered a standard of care to prevent CI-AKI. Isotonic saline and sodium bicarbonate were found equally effective and superior to hypotonic fluids. Isotonic saline is preferred, however, because it is less expensive and does not have to be compound. There is no clear evidence from the literature to guide the choice of the optimal rate and duration of fluid infusion in CI-AKI prevention, but most studies suggest that the fluids should be started at least 1 hour before and continued for 3 hours to 6 hours after contrast-media administration. A good urine output (>150 mL/h) in the 6 hours after the procedure has been associated with reduced rates of AKI.[30] Central venous pressure (CVP)-guided IV hydration was evaluated versus standard hydration in a prospective, randomized, double-blinded, comparative analysis in patients with CKD and heart failure. The study showed 46% decrease in CI-AKI in the CVP-guided IV hydration group compared with the standard hydration group. The rate of fluid administration was guided by CVP as follows: 3 mL/kg/h for CVP less than 6 cm H_2O, 1.5 mL/kg/h for CVP 6 cm H_2O to 12 cm H_2O, and 1 mL/kg/h for CVP greater than 12 cm H_2O. The standard hydration group received 1 mL/kg/h. The IV infusion rate was dynamically adjusted according to the level of CVP per hour during hydration and was maintained for 6 hours preprocedural and 12 hours post-procedural. The CVP-guided hydration group received significantly higher overall fluids volume with no significant increase in heart failure exacerbations.[31]

Another effective strategy to prevent CI-AKI is the use of the RenalGuard system (PLC Medical Systems, Franklin, Massachusetts), which includes using IV isotonic fluids bolus followed by a dose of loop diuretic an hour before contrast administration. Subsequently, the system measures the patient urine output in real time during the procedure to infuse equal volume of isotonic fluids in order to dilute the contrast media and forces diuresis to minimize contrast toxicity and contact time with the glomeruli. The use of the RenalGuard system significantly reduced rates of CI-AKI compared with standard volume expansion and also was associated with decreased rates of death, dialysis, and major cardiovascular event.[32]

Along with adequate hydration, using the least necessary contrast volume is essential to prevent CI-AKI. Contrast volume and CI-AKI have a linear relationship. According to a retrospective analysis of the Mayo Clinic Percutaneous Intervention Registry, there is 12% risk increase of CI-AKI for every 100 mL of contrast used.[33]

Minimizing contrast volume can be achieved by using a contrast reduction system instead of manual contrast injection. Multiple studies have showed that using contrast reduction system is safe, can maintain the image quality, and provides an additional tool to prevent CI-AKI by minimizing total contrast volume.[34,35]

Further minimization or elimination of iodinated contrast volume can be done by using CO_2 angiography, which has been used in patients who have very high risk of developing CI-AKI. In a systematic review, however, CO_2 use did not significantly reduce the rate of AKI. Furthermore, when CO_2 was used as primary imaging agent, AKI average incidence

still remained relatively elevated at 6.2%. As well, the technique requires meticulous attention to detail because it is associated relatively high incidence of nonrenal adverse side effects.[36]

Further details about contrast-induced nephropathy re discussed in more specifics later.

PROGNOSTIC IMPACT OF CHRONIC KIDNEY DISEASE ON PERIPHERAL ARTERIAL DISEASE OUTCOMES: MORTALITY, AMPUTATION, AND REPEAT REVASCULARIZATION

It is essential to recognize that CKD not only is a risk factor for PAD but also an important predictor of poor outcomes. Patients with CKD and PAD have worse overall outcome, including overall complications, revascularization success rate, and mortality. Data have been controversial regarding the impact of CKD on amputation rate. Table 1 summarizes the prognostic studies.

In a retrospective analysis on CLI patients, to determine the impact of severe CKD (stages 4 and 5) on infra-inguinal PVI outcome, 879 PVIs were analyzed from January 2002 through December 2009. Severe CKD was present in 125 (14%) and increased the risk of late mortality hazard ratio ([HR] 2.4; 95% CI, 1.8–3.2; $P<.01$), amputation (HR 2.1; 95% CI, 1.1–3.9; P [0.02]), and death or amputation (HR 1.8; 95% CI, 1.3–2.4; P [0.04]), without increasing the risk of late reinterventions or major adverse limb events (MALEs).[37]

CKD predicted worse short-term mortality (HR 2.84; 95% CI, 1.265–2.103), amputation rate, and overall MALE-free survival (HR 1.6 [2.026–3.990]) in symptomatic PAD and CLI patients who underwent PVI, compared with normal renal function patients. There was no significant difference in the PVI technical success rate between the 2 groups.[38]

The 1-year mortality of a CKD patient who has a GFR less than 30 mL/min and presents with gangrene can be as high as 44%. This statistic almost approaches the reported rates for elderly patients who have renal insufficiency and are treated for decompensated heart failure and acute MI. These data were derived from a large, national cohort of male veterans who received an initial diagnosis of CLI, in whom the presence of renal insufficiency was a strong, and for whom independent risk factor for mortality within 1 year.[39]

In a retrospective study that reviewed 1010 hospitalized PAD patients (15.5% had CKD)

Table 1 Summary of prognostic studies of peripheral artery disease in chronic kidney disease patients		
Study	**Chronic Kidney Disease Patients**	**Prognosis Specific to Chronic Kidney Disease**
Impact of CKD stage 4/5 on infra-inguinal PVI outcome[37]	14% of 879 PVIs	MALE (OR 2.8; 95% CI, 1.3–6.1) Mortality (HR 2.4; 95% CI, 1.8–3.2) Amputation (HR 2.1; 95% CI, 1.1–3 .9)
Effect of CKD on clinical outcome post-PVI[38]	10% of 2739 patients	MALE (HR 1.6; 95% CI, 2.026–3.990) Mortality (HR 2.84; 95% CI, 1.265–2.103)
Impact of CKD on mortality in PAD[39]	71% of 5787 patients	Mortality CKD stage 3 (OR 1.3; 95% CI, 1.13–1.52) CKD stage 5 (OR 3.2; 95% CI, 2.61–4.02)
CKD and the short-term risk of mortality and amputation in hospitalized patient with PAD[5]	15.5% of 1010 patients	Amputation CKD stage 3 (HR 1.06; 95% CI, 0.73–1.55) CKD stages 4–5 (HR 1.47; 95% CI, 0.97–2.21) Mortality CKD stage 3 (HR 1.56; 95% CI, 1.03–2.37) CKD stages 4–5 (HR 2.53; 95% CI, 1.62–3.97)
Impact of CKD on PVI of Femoropopliteal arterial disease[41]	55% of 440 patients	Amputation CKD stages 3b–4 (HR 1.6; 95% CI, 0.95–2.6) CKD stage 5 (HR 4.1; 95% CI, 2.5–6.8) Mortality CKD stages 3b–4 (HR 2.8; 95% CI, 2.0–4.1) CKD stage 5 (HR 5.7; 95% CI, 3.7–8.9)
Revascularization vs medical therapy survival in patients with CKD and CLI[42]	56% of 351 patients	AFS CKD stage 3 (HR 0.51; 95% CI, 0.29–0.99) CKD stages 4–5 (HR 0.44; 95% CI, 0.17–1.14) Overall survival CKD stage 3 (HR 0.51; 95% CI, 0.29–0.99) CKD stages 4–5 (HR 0.33; 95% CI, 0.12–0.91)
CKD and acute and long-term outcome of patients with PAD and CLI[40]	20% of 41,882 patients	Amputation CKD stage 2 (HR 0.99; 95% CI, 0.91–1.09) CKD stage 3 (HR 1.03; 95% CI, 0.96–1.11) CKD stage 4 (HR 1.08; 95% CI, 0.96–1.22) CKD stage 5 (HR 1.43; 95% CI, 1.31–1.55) Mortality CKD stage 2 (HR 1.17; 95% CI, 1.09–1.26)

(continued on next page)

Study	Chronic Kidney Disease Patients	Prognosis Specific to Chronic Kidney Disease
		CKD stage 3 (HR 1.26; 95% CI, 1.19–1.34) CKD stage 4 (HR 1.74; 95% CI, 1.59–1.91) CKD stage 5 (HR 5 2.59; 95% CI, 2.41–2.78)
Effect of CKD on mortality in patients who had PVI[44]	27% of 755 patients	5-y mortality HR 1.57; 95% CI, 1.13–2.19

from May 2004 to January 2009, patients were classified into 4 groups according to the GFR (Fig. 4). CKD was an independent predictor of 1-year mortality in hospitalized PAD patients due to ALI or CLI. The mortality rates also were worse among CKD patients based on the CKD stage (stages 4-5 vs stages 1-3). CKD, however, was not an independent predictor of limb amputation.[5]

The worsening of prognosis per the degree of renal impairment was found significant in another study correspondingly; however, the impact of CKD on the amputation rate was controversial. In a large cohort study, including 41,882 patients with PAD who had an index hospitalization between January 1, 2009, and December 31, 2011, CKD patients underwent significantly fewer revascularizations (0.9-fold fewer; P<.001); had a nearly 2-fold higher amputation rate (P<.001); and had a nearly 3-fold higher in-hospital mortality rate (P<.001) compared with patients with normal kidney function (Fig. 5).[40]

As well, advanced CKD was a predictor of higher amputation rates in a retrospective study on diabetic patients undergoing endovascular treatment of femoropopliteal disease due to claudication or CLI (HR 4.1; 95% CI, 2.5–6.8). Furthermore, CKD patients had higher rates of all-cause mortality, major acute limb events, and postoperative death.[41]

Despite the poor prognosis associated with CKD in CLI patients, revascularization procedure improved prognosis compared with conservative therapy. In an intention-to-treat cohort study, Ortmann and colleagues[42] reviewed a population of 383 CLI patients for 12 months. Moderate to severe CKD patients had worse overall survival, amputation-free survival (AFS), and limb salvage rate compared with patient with mild CKD or normal kidney function. As well, patients who received revascularization regardless of any level of renal impairment and had better overall survival compared with patients who had medical therapy and/or amputation.

Specific risk factors were determined to predict mortality in CKD patients who are undergoing a peripheral revascularization:

1. Age greater than 80 years old
2. Coronary artery disease
3. Chronic obstructive pulmonary disease
4. Dependent preoperative ambulation status
5. Rest pain/tissue loss

The presence of 3 or more risk factors resulted in a predicted 1-year mortality of 64%. According to a regional multicenter registry review, from 2003 to 2013 for dialysis patients presenting with CLI (90%) and claudication (8%). Open surgical bypass was performed to 70% of the patients and 30% underwent endovascular intervention. Overall survival rate at 5 years remained low at 21%. Overall 2-year AFS rate was 17%. In this study, the survival, AFS, and freedom from MALE outcomes did not differ

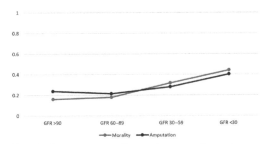

Fig. 4. One-year mortality and amputation rate per GFR group in hospitalized patients due to PAD (P<.006). (Adapted from Lacroix, Philippe et al. Chronic kidney disease and the short-term risk of mortality and amputation in patients hospitalized for peripheral artery disease. Journal of Vascular Surgery, Volume 58, Issue 4, 966 – 97; with permission.)

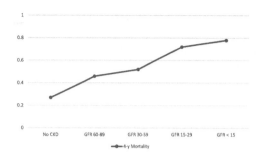

Fig. 5. Four-year mortality rate per GFR group (*P*<.001). (*Adapted from* Florian Luders., et al. CKD and Acute and Long-Term Outcome of Patients with Peripheral Artery Disease and Critical Limb Ischemia. CJASN Feb 2016;11(2):216-22; with permission.)

significantly between revascularization techniques. At 2 years, endovascular patency was higher than open bypass (76% vs 26%; 95% CI, 0.28–0.71; *P* [0.02]).[43]

Parallel to the impact on short-term outcome, CKD predicted poor long-term outcome. PAD patients with CKD had worse 5-year mortality compared with non-CKD patients. In a retrospective study on claudication and CLI patients at a Veteran Affairs hospital, 755 patients who had a PVI were reviewed. The presence of CKD in 204 patients was associated with decreased survival (5-year survival probability of CKD compared with non-CKD [HR 1.57; 95% CI, 1.13–2.19]).[44]

Additional factors to improve survival and AFS in CKD patients presenting with CLI were investigated. The pedal arch patency was a potential modifiable factor, because it showed impact on the rate and time of wound healing in some studies. The impact of the pedal arch patency on survival and AFS in below-the-knee angioplasty were assessed in a prospective study that included 32 ERSD patients on hemodialysis with CLI and consecutive infrapopliteal angioplasty over a 5-year period, 2010 to 2014. A total of 44 vessels in 32 ischemic legs was treated. The 1 and 2 years AFS rates were 56% and 34% respectively. The pedal arch quality had no impact on the predefined endpoints. The 30-day mortality was only 6%, with only 11 patients requiring a redo procedure. These findings emphasize the feasibility and safety of endovascular approach in these highly multimorbid patients.[45]

SUMMARY

In summary, renal impairment patients are at an increased risk of developing PAD. They require close monitoring and screening for PAD, particularly those who reach ESRD. A normal ABI should be followed by further studies, such as TBI and/or exercise treadmill ABI when clinical suspicion is high. When an imaging study is indicated, invasive angiography should be considered first because it offers opportunity to intervene. Technical challenges and complications during angioplasty are more common in CKD patients due to increased vascular calcifications and the risk of CI-AKI. When indicated, however, angioplasty using CI-AKI preventive measures is safer than surgical bypass, particularly in high-risk patients, and offers better overall outcome, including quality of life, AFS, and survival, compared with conservative management. Prognosis overall is poor compared with non-CKD patients and gets worse with advanced renal impairment stages. Prevention by treating risk factors and early diagnosis are key elements to improving outcome.

DISCLOSURE

The authors have nothing to disclose.

REFERENCES

1. Payne MM. Charles Theodore Dotter. The father of intervention. Tex Heart Inst J 2001;28(1):28–38.
2. Shu J, Santulli G. Update on peripheral artery disease: epidemiology and evidence-based facts. Atherosclerosis 2018;275:379–81.
3. Creager MA, Belkin M, Bluth EI, et al. 2012 ACCF/AHA/ACR/SCAI/SIR/STS/SVM/SVN/SVS Key Data Elements and Definitions for Peripheral Atherosclerotic Vascular Disease. J Am Coll Cardiol 2012; 59(3):294–357.
4. CDC. Peripheral arterial disease fact sheet 06/16/2016. Available at: https://www.cdc.gov/dhdsp/data_statistics/fact_sheets/fs_pad.htm. Accessed September 24, 2019.
5. Lacroix P, Aboyans V, Desormais I, et al. Chronic kidney disease and the short-term risk of mortality and amputation in patients hospitalized for peripheral artery disease. J Vasc Surg 2013;58(4):966–71.
6. Herzog CA, Asinger RW, Berger AK, et al. Cardiovascular disease in chronic kidney disease. A clinical update from Kidney Disease: Improving Global Outcomes (KDIGO). Kidney Int 2011;80(6): 572–86.
7. Gerhard-Herman MD, Gornik HL, Barrett C, et al. 2016 AHA/ACC Guideline on the Management of Patients With Lower Extremity Peripheral Artery Disease: Executive Summary: A Report of the American College of Cardiology/American Heart

Association Task Force on Clinical Practice Guidelines. Circulation 2017;135:e686–725.

8. Selvin E, Erlinger TP. Prevalence of and risk factors for peripheral arterial disease in the United States. Results from the National Health and Nutrition Examination Survey, 1999–2000. Circulation 2004;110: 738–43.

9. Garimella PS, Hirsch AT. Peripheral artery disease and chronic kidney disease: clinical synergy to improve outcomes. Adv Chronic Kidney Dis 2014; 21(6):460–71.

10. Ašćerić RR, Dimković NB, Trajković GŽ, et al. Prevalence, clinical characteristics, and predictors of peripheral arterial disease in hemodialysis patients: a cross-sectional study. BMC Nephrol 2019;20(1):281.

11. Baber U, Mann D, Shimbo D, et al. Combined role of reduced estimated glomerular filtration rate and microalbuminuria on the prevalence of peripheral arterial disease. Am J Cardiol 2009;104(10): 1446–51.

12. Arinze NV, Gregory A, Francis JM, et al. Unique aspects of peripheral artery disease in patients with chronic kidney disease. Vasc Med 2019;24(3): 251–60.

13. Kobayashi S. Cardiovascular events in chronic kidney disease (CKD)—an importance of vascular calcification and microcirculatory impairment. Ren Replace Ther 2016;2:55.

14. Ho CY, Shanahan CM. Medial Arterial Calcification. An Overlooked Player in Peripheral Arterial Disease. Arterioscler Thromb Vasc Biol 2016;36:1475–82.

15. National Kidney Foundation 2010. Vascular Dysfunction atherosclerosis and calcification. Insight and implication in Chronic Kidney Disease. Available at: https://www.kidney.org/sites/default/files/12-10-0210_LBA_Vascular_bklt_LowRes.pdf. November 16, 2019.

16. Brodmann M, Werner M, Brinton TJ, et al. Safety and Performance of Lithoplasty for Treatment of Calcified Peripheral Artery Lesions. J Am Coll Cardiol 2017;70(7):908–10.

17. Gradman WS, Cohen W, Haji-Aghaii M. Arteriovenous fistula construction in the thigh with transposed superficial femoral vein: Our initial experience. J Vasc Surg 2001;33(5):968–75.

18. Okamoto S, Iida O, Mano T. Current perspective on hemodialysis patients with peripheral artery disease. Ann Vasc Dis 2017;10(2):88–91.

19. Rooke TW, Hirsch AT, Misra S, et al. 2011 ACCF/AHA focused update of the guideline for the management of patients with peripheral artery disease (updating the 2005 guideline): a report of the American College of Cardiology Foundation/American Heart Association Task Force on practice guidelines. J Am Coll Cardiol 2011;58(19):2020–45.

20. Bradbury AW, Adam DJ, Bell J, et al. Bypass versus Angioplasty in Severe Ischaemia of the Leg (BASIL) trial: An intention-to-treat analysis of amputation-free and overall survival in patients randomized to a bypass surgery-first or a balloon angioplasty-first revascularization strategy. J Vasc Surg 2010;51(5):5S–17S.

21. Nishibe T, Kondo Y, Dardik A, et al. Stent placement in the superficial femoral artery for patients on chronic hemodialysis with peripheral artery disease. Int Angiol 2009;28(6):484–9.

22. Meyer A, Lang W, Borowski M, et al. In-hospital outcomes in patients with critical limb ischemia and end-stage renal disease after revascularization. J Vasc Surg 2016;63(4):966–73.

23. Garimella PS, Balakrishnan P, Correa A, et al. Nationwide Trends in Hospital Outcomes and Utilization After Lower Limb Revascularization in Patients on Hemodialysis. JACC Cardiovasc Intervention 2017;10(20):2101–10.

24. O'Hare AM, Bertenthal D, Sidawy AN, et al. Renal insufficiency and use of revascularization among a national cohort of men with advanced lower extremity peripheral arterial disease. Clin J Am Soc Nephrol 2006;1(2):297–304.

25. Kumada Y, Aoyama T, Ishii H, et al. Long-term outcome of percutaneous transluminal angioplasty in chronic haemodialysis patients with peripheral arterial disease. Nephrol Dial Transplant 2008; 23(12):3996–4001.

26. Gilmore D, Dib M, Evenson A, et al. Endovascular management of critical limb ischemia in renal transplant patients. Ann Vasc Surg 2014;28(1):159–63.

27. Prasad A, Hughston H, Michalek J, et al. Acute kidney injury in patients undergoing endovascular therapy for critical limb ischemia. Catheter Cardiovasc Interv 2019;94:636–41.

28. Lautin EM, Freeman NJ, Schoenfeld AH, et al. Radiocontrast-associated renal dysfunction: incidence and risk factors. Am J Roentgenol 1991; 157(1):49–58.

29. Prasad A, Ortiz-Lopez C, Khan A, et al. Acute kidney injury following peripheral angiography and endovascular therapy: A systematic review of the literature. Catheter Cardiovasc Interv 2016;88: 264–73.

30. Kidney Disease: Improving Global Outcomes (KDIGO) Acute Kidney Injury Work Group. KDIGO Clinical Practice Guideline for Acute Kidney Injury. Kidney inter 2012;2(Suppl):1–138.

31. Qian G, Fu Z, Guo J, et al. Prevention of contrast-induced nephropathy by central venous pressure–guided fluid administration in chronic kidney disease and congestive heart failure patients. JACC Cardiovasc Intervention 2016;9(1):89–96.

32. Mattathil S, Ghumman S, Weinerman J, et al. Use of the RenalGuard system to prevent contrast-induced AKI: A meta-analysis. J Interv Cardiol 2017;30:480–7.

33. Rihal CS, Textor SC, Grill DE, et al. Incidence and prognostic importance of acute renal failure after percutaneous coronary intervention. Circulation 2002;105(19):2259–64.

34. Gurm HS, Mavromatis K, Bertolet B, et al. Minimizing radiographic contrast administration during coronary angiography using a novel contrast reduction system: A multicenter observational study of the DyeVert™ plus contrast reduction system. Catheter Cardiovasc Interv 2019;93:1228–35.

35. Corcione N, Biondi-Zoccai G, Ferraro P, et al. Dye-Vert Plus System for Contrast Reduction and Real-Time Monitoring During Coronary and Peripheral Procedures: First Experience. J Invasive Cardiol 2017;29(8):259–62.

36. Ghumman SS, Weinerman J, Khan A, et al. Contrast induced-acute kidney injury following peripheral angiography with carbon dioxide versus iodinated contrast media: A meta-analysis and systematic review of current literature. Catheter Cardiovasc Interv 2017;90:437–48.

37. Patel VI, Mukhopadhyay S, Guest JM, et al. Impact of severe chronic kidney disease on outcomes of infrainguinal peripheral arterial intervention. J Vasc Surg 2014;59(2):368–75.

38. Kim HO, Kim JM, Woo JS, et al. Effects of chronic kidney disease on clinical outcomes in patients with peripheral artery disease undergoing endovascular treatment: Analysis from the K-VIS ELLA registry. Int J Cardiol 2018;262:32–7.

39. O'Hare AM, Bertenthal D, Shlipak MG, et al. Impact of Renal Insufficiency on Mortality in Advanced Lower Extremity Peripheral Arterial Disease. J Am Soc Nephrol 2005;16(2):514–9.

40. Lüders F, Bunzemeier H, Engelbertz C, et al. CKD and acute and long-term outcome of patients with peripheral artery disease and critical limb ischemia. Clin J Am Soc Nephrol 2016;11(2):216–22.

41. Heideman PP, Rajebi MR, McKusick MA, et al. Impact of chronic kidney disease on clinical outcomes of endovascular treatment for femoropopliteal arterial disease. J Vasc Interv Radiol 2016;27(8):1204–14.

42. Ortmann J, Gahl B, Diehm N, et al. Survival benefits of revascularization in patients with critical limb ischemia and renal insufficiency. J Vasc Surg 2012;56(3):737–45.e1.

43. Fallon JM, Goodney PP, Stone DH, et al. Outcomes of lower extremity revascularization among the hemodialysis-dependent. J Vasc Surg 2015;62(5):1183–91.e1.

44. Xie JX, Glorioso TJ, Dattilo PB, et al. Effect of chronic kidney disease on mortality in patients who underwent lower extremity peripheral vascular intervention. Am J Cardiol 2017;119(4):669–74.

45. Meyer A, Schinz K, Lang W, et al. Outcomes and influence of the pedal arch in below-the-knee angioplasty in patients with end-stage renal disease and critical limb ischemia. Ann Vasc Surg 2016;35:121–9.

Implications of Renal Disease in Patients Undergoing Structural Interventions

Vinayak Nagaraja, MBBS, MS, MMed (Clin Epi), FRACP,
Samir Kapadia, MD*

KEYWORDS

- Severe valvular heart disease • Transcatheter valve interventions • End-stage renal disease

---

KEY POINTS

- Prevalence of calcific valvular heart disease in patients with renal dysfunction is high and is an independent predictor of cardiovascular mortality.
- End-stage renal disease patients experience higher rates of major bleeding and major vascular complications after transfemoral transcatheter aortic valve replacement.
- A multidisciplinary team approach that includes a renal physician when managing patients with chronic kidney disease and severe valvular heart disease.
- Acute kidney injury after transcatheter valve intervention carries a poor prognosis.
- Measures to prevent acute kidney injury need to be undertaken.

INTRODUCTION

The prevalence of calcific valvular heart disease (VHD) in patients with renal dysfunction is high.[1] The mortality rates at 5 years for patients with renal dysfunction and severe valvular heart disease (severe aortic stenosis, mitral regurgitation) are twice those of the normal population.[1] Cardiac valve calcification is an independent predictor of cardiovascular mortality in peritoneal dialysis patients[2] and transcatheter valve interventions are an attractive alternative to invasive surgery in patients with chronic kidney disease (CKD) and severe VHD who often have multiple comorbidities.[3–5] This review aims to summarize the epidemiology, pathophysiology, and impact of transcatheter valve interventions in patients with VHD and CKD.

EPIDEMIOLOGY

The first manifestation of renal insufficiency-induced VHD is calcification, and aortic valve calcification increases with decreasing estimated glomerular filtration rate.[6,7] On echocardiography, valvular calcification can be detected in around 35% to 40% of patients with end-stage renal disease (ESRD).[8,9] In individuals with ESRD the prevalence of VHD is higher and is 14% in hemodialysis patients and 12% in peritoneal dialysis patients.[10] This risk is lowered to 7.4% after renal transplantation.[10] Aortic stenosis is the most common VHD among patients with ESRD and its prevalence ranges between 6% and 13%.[6] The odds of developing of significant aortic stenosis in the long term is higher in patients with CKD and the progression is accelerated by advancing renal disease.[1] The progression of aortic stenosis is twice as fast in patients with CKD ($0.2 \text{ cm}^2/\text{y}$) when compared with the normal population ($0.1 \text{ cm}^2/\text{y}$).[6,11] Increasing age, malnutrition, inflammation, higher phosphate levels, calcium phosphorus product, and vitamin D levels, and duration of dialysis are

---

Department of Cardiovascular Medicine, Cleveland Clinic Foundation, 9500 Euclid Avenue, Cleveland, OH 44195, USA
* Corresponding author.
E-mail address: kapadis@ccf.org

independent predictors of aortic valve calcification/stenosis.[12–14]

PATHOPHYSIOLOGY

The pathophysiology of VHD in patients with CKD is multifaceted and complex. Valve calcification is a result of metabolic and hemodynamic factors. From a metabolic perspective parathyroid hormone, beta 2-microglobulin hyperphosphatemia, and calcium phosphate product play an important role in interstitial cell calcification in the valve leaflets. These elements result in abnormal calcium and phosphate metabolism.[12] Hypovitaminosis D can lead to vascular calcification,[15] and progression of aortic stenosis is due to secondary hyperparathyroidism.[16] In rabbit models hypervitaminosis D results in aortic valve calcification.[17] Amyloid deposition also contributes to aortic valve calcification.[18] Fig. 1 summarizes the pathophysiology of valvular calcification. Vitamin K antagonists are linked aortic, vascular, and coronary calcification in patients undergoing hemodialysis.[19–21] From a hemodynamic standpoint, congenital conditions, such as bicuspid aortic valves, accelerate aortic valve calcification.[22] The increased shear stress results in the initiation and progression of aortic valve calcification. The synergistic relationship between valve calcification/progression and the arteriovenous fistula is unclear. The volume overload as a result of arteriovenous fistula results in cardiac chamber enlargement and aggravates mitral and tricuspid regurgitation. Furthermore, the creation of a new arteriovenous fistula could potentially lead to decompensated cardiac failure.[23] Mitral valve regurgitation could be partially/completely functional as a result of annular dilatation, left atrial dilation, or volume overload.[24] Mitral annular calcification (MAC) has a similar pathophysiology to aortic valve calcification.[25–27] Patients with ESRD have extensive MAC, commonly resulting in mixed mitral valve disease/mitral stenosis. These patients are also prone to endocarditis and atrial arrythmias.

IMAGING CONSIDERATIONS SPECIFIC TO CHRONIC KIDNEY DISEASE

Symptomatic VHD in patients with CKD can be confounded by anemia and frailty, and hence echocardiographic assessment is crucial. Mitral valve regurgitation is often worsened with uncontrolled hypertension and volume status. It is best to perform echocardiography after dialysis with good blood pressure control. Theoretically,

one would speculate that this would improve the accuracy of echocardiographic parameters for left ventricular mass, systolic/diastolic function, and pulmonary pressure; however, there is not enough evidence to support this.[28] Large body habitus in patients with CKD can lead to suboptimal imaging windows and make Doppler beam alignment difficult. Septal hypertrophy as a result of long-standing hypertension is a common comorbidity in patients with CKD, which makes calculation of left ventricular outflow tract (LVOT) area tricky. The arteriovenous fistula results in a high output state and leads to overestimation of transvalvular gradients. Hence, temporary arteriovenous fistula compression[29] can lead to more accurate estimation of transvalvular gradients. Paradoxic low-flow/low-gradient severe aortic stenosis is an entity common in elderly hypertensive individuals alongside heart failure with preserved ejection fraction.[30] A dimensionless severity index of less than 0.25 indicates severe aortic stenosis and should be used more often than aortic valve area.[31] This index is less variable, and more reproducible compared with aortic valve area, and has prognostic consequences.[31–33] Cardiac computerized tomography (cardiac CT) has revolutionized the preoperative assessment of severe aortic stenosis (AS) in the era of transcatheter aortic valve replacement (TAVR). Cardiac CT provides important information, such as annulus measurement, calcium distribution coronary ostia, vascular anatomy, and the feasibility of TAVR. An aortic valve calcium score of ≥2000 Agatston units in men and ≥1200 in women is diagnostic of severe AS.[34] This is especially helpful in complex patients in whom there is a diagnostic dilemma, such as discordant severe calcified aortic valve disease.[34,35] To prevent contrast nephropathy in patients with CKD, noncontrast cardiac magnetic resonance imaging (CMRI) is useful to assess the annulus,[36] although CMRI is limited with regard to visualization of calcification.[36] Another contrast-sparing option is transesophageal echocardiography.[37]

TRANSCATHETER AORTIC VALVE REPLACEMENT OUTCOMES IN INDIVIDUALS WITH RENAL DYSFUNCTION

Aortic valve disease is the most common VHD in individuals with end-stage renal disease.[38] The mortality after surgical aortic valve replacement is nearly 20%[39,40] in individuals on dialysis, and is as high as 50% in elderly dialysis patients.[41] TAVR has become the standard of care in

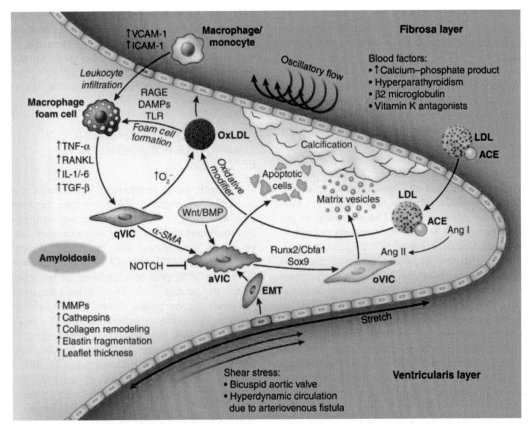

Fig. 1. Pathophysiology of calcified aortic valve disease. (*From* Marwick TH, Amann K, Bangalore S, et al. Chronic kidney disease and valvular heart disease: conclusions from a Kidney Disease: Improving Global Outcomes (KDIGO) Controversies Conference. *Kidney international.* 2019;96(4):836-849; with permission.)

individuals with severe AS, with robust survival benefit and symptom relief.[42–47] Hence, TAVR seems to be an attractive percutaneous option with a shorter length of hospital stay.[48] However, patients with advanced CKD are traditionally excluded from randomized trials. The evidence in this regard is mostly from retrospective studies, which are prone to selection bias.

A meta-analysis reported the outcomes of TAVR in 3500 patients with end-stage renal disease.[49] The mean STS score was more than 10 in most studies. Individuals with renal failure had a 30-day mortality rate of 10%, whereas at 1 year the mortality rate was 33%. Bleeding was prevalent in 17% of patients; 14% of individuals had a permanent pacemaker implantation and 7% suffered a major vascular complication. The largest meta-analysis so far,[50] of 12 studies with more than 40,000 patients with CKD, suggested a higher short-term (1 month) overall mortality (risk ratio [RR] = 1.56; 95% CI, 1.34–1.80), long-term cardiovascular mortality (RR = 1.44; 95% CI, 1.22–1.70) and overall mortality (RR = 1.66; 95% CI, 1.45–1.91) compared with non-

CKD patients. From a procedural standpoint, permanent pacemaker rates (RR =1.20; 95% CI, 1.03–1.39) and major bleeding (RR = 1.60; 95% CI, 1.26–2.02) were higher in CKD compared with non-CKD patients. A meta-regression analysis demonstrated that mortality and periprocedural complications increased with advanced CKD.

The largest study to date that compared TAVR outcomes between ESRD with nondialysis patients comes from the transcatheter valve therapies (TVT) registry.[51] This TVT registry analysis consists of more than 3000 patients with ESRD on dialysis, and these patients were younger, and more likely to be African American, multimorbid, with higher STS score, compared with the nondialysis patients. They were also found to have a higher prevalence of concomitant moderate to severe mitral regurgitation, tricuspid regurgitation, and poor left ventricular systolic function. The ESRD cohort were more likely to undergo TAVR on an urgent basis with lower utilization of the transfemoral approach presumably due to severe peripheral

vascular disease. Individuals with ESRD experienced substantially higher in-hospital mortality (5.1% vs 3.4%; $P<.01$) and 1-year mortality (hazard ratio = 1.28; 95% CI, 1.17–1.41). Higher rates of major bleeding and major vascular complications were observed in patients with ESRD undergoing transfemoral TAVR. Patients with ESRD had similar incidence of stroke to non-CKD patients. However, a longer length of stay was observed in the ESRD cohort.

Some of the reasons that patients with ESRD/CKD have worse outcomes include platelet dysfunction, anemia of chronic disease, severe peripheral vascular disease, and frailty, with multiple other comorbidities. The mortality in patients with CKD seems to have decreased in these studies over time.[52–56] This is probably because of better expertise/training, operator/center volume, and device technology given that these studies are retrospective and observational selection bias is highly likely. With an aging community with multiple comorbidities, patient selection is key and identifying the markers of futility is crucial. Allende and colleagues[52] assessed TAVR outcomes in patients with ESRD with atrial fibrillation. The mortality rate at 2 years was 100%, implying that TAVR is futile in individuals with patients with ESRD with atrial fibrillation. Other markers of futility include frailty, concomitant severe mitral regurgitation, severe pulmonary hypertension, and oxygen-dependent chronic lung disease.[57] TAVR as a bridge to renal transplant is rarely performed,[58] although it offers new hope to patients with a progressive eventually fatal disease, such as ESRD. It is currently challenging to identify patients with ESRD who would gain the survival benefit from TAVR.

TRANSCATHETER AORTIC VALVE REPLACEMENT IN RENAL TRANSPLANT RECIPIENTS

Renal transplantation has improved the quality of life and survival in patients with ESRD.[59] This is a special group of patients with CKD and with improved survival they eventually need management of VHD. Only two studies have explored the role of TAVR in kidney transplant recipients.[60,61] The largest study[60] so far consists of 72 kidney transplant recipients. This retrospective study compared TAVR outcomes in kidney transplant recipients with individuals with native kidneys and comparable kidney function. Renal function declined in the kidney transplant recipients and the need for long-term renal replacement therapy was higher (hazard ratio =

2.09, 95% CI, 1.03–3.86) with most of them initiated periprocedurally. Nevertheless, mortality was not significantly different among the groups. Consideration should be given to referring complex patients with CKD to high-volume centers and operators to achieve better outcomes.[62]

ACUTE KIDNEY INJURY AFTER TRANSCATHETER AORTIC VALVE REPLACEMENT

The prevalence of severe renal impairment in individuals undergoing TAVR ranges between 29% and 34%.[63,64] Contrast-induced nephropathy continues to be a major concern after interventional procedures. The incidence of acute kidney injury (AKI) after TAVR varies between 8.3% and 58%, probably because of heterogenous definitions.[65–68] The Valve Academic Research Consortium-2 (VARC2) criteria[69] are currently used for diagnosing AKI (Table 1). AKI after TAVR is a poor prognostic sign.[70,71] A 5- to 8-fold increase in 30-day mortality after TAVR is observed when complicated by AKI. At 12 months, the mortality is at least 3 times higher compared with individuals without AKI.[67,70,72] AKI is linked to longer length of stay and greater intensive care utilization, adding to the economic burden on health care.[73] Long-term hemodialysis incidence was as high as 21% resulting in an inferior quality of life.[67,70,72]

AKI after TAVR is multifaceted and the mechanism is poorly understood. It is probably an amalgamation of predisposing conditions and intraprocedural events. The most important risk factor for AKI after TAVR is poor baseline creatinine clearance.[74] Predisposing risk factors that are independent predictors of AKI include preprocedural New York Heart Association class IV, cardiogenic shock, urgent/emergent TAVR, higher stage of CKD, anemia needing blood transfusion, nephrotoxic drugs, past medical history of hypertension, peripheral vascular disease, heart failure, atrial fibrillation, diabetes, chronic obstructive pulmonary disease, and cerebrovascular accident.[75–79] Periprocedural insults can occur as a result of rapid ventricular pacing during valve deployment, intraoperative hypotension, general anesthesia, major bleeding, cholesterol embolization due to equipment manipulation, hypovolemic shock, and paravalvular aortic regurgitation.[78,80–82] The combination of prerenal azotemia and nephrotoxic influences results in acute tubular necrosis. A bedside risk score[83] was developed

Table 1
Valve Academic Research Consortium-2 criteria for acute kidney injury

Stage	Serum Creatinine (sCr)	Urine Output
1	Increase in sCr to 150%–199% (1.5–1.99× increase compared with baseline) OR increase of ≥0.3 mg/dL (≥26.4 mmol/L)	<0.5 mL/kg/h for >6 but <12 h
2	<0.3 mL/kg/h for ≥24 h OR anuria for ≥12 h	<0.5 mL/kg/h for >12 but <24 h
3	Increase in sCr to ≥300% (>3× increase compared with baseline) OR sCr of ≥4.0 mg/dL (≥354 mmol/L) with an acute increase of ≥0.5 mg/dL (44 mmol/L)	<0.3 mL/kg/h for ≥24 h OR anuria for ≥12 h

From Kappetein AP, Head SJ, Genereux P, et al. Updated standardized endpoint definitions for transcatheter aortic valve implantation: the Valve Academic Research Consortium-2 consensus document. *European heart journal.* 2012;33(19):2403-2418; with permission.

to predict AKI after TAVR that includes New York Heart Association class IV, hemoglobin, alternate access TAVR, valve-in-valve TAVR, creatinine clearance, and body weight (kg). This score has a c-statistic of 0.73 and can be a useful bedside tool.

A multidisciplinary team approach should be used when managing patients with CKD and severe VHD. The team should include a renal physician, and optimization of predisposing factors as mentioned above should be undertaken. Maintenance of euvolemic status and cessation of nephrotoxins before TAVR is crucial.[84] AKI depends on the contrast dose administered[70] and minimizing contrast use is important. Low-osmolar contrast agents prove to be of benefit in these circumstances.[85] Apart from intravenous crystalloids, sodium bicarbonate and N-acetyl-cysteine infusions have not been proven to reduce AKI.[86,87] Newer devices in the market, such as the RenalGuard System, have shown some promise.[68,88] This device provides furosemide-induced diuresis complemented with isotonic intravenous hydration and has been proved to be an effective prevention strategy in PROTECT-TAVI trial.[68] Intraoperatively, avoiding predilatation, use of local/conscious sedation, and reducing the duration of rapid pacing are other useful strategies to prevent hypotension. A self-expanding TAVR device can be considered in patients with CKD to avoid rapid pacing; however, there is no evidence to support this hypothesis.[89] There are some limitations of the VARC2 criteria that can be potentially addressed in future definitions. It does not address temporary or permanent renal replacement as a separate stage and the use of urine output in day-to-day practice is challenging. In addition, assessment of creatinine beyond 48 hours is difficult due to early discharge. **Fig. 2** captures the predisposing factors for post-TAVR AKI and potential prevention strategies.

TRANSCATHETER MITRAL VALVE INTERVENTION

Mitral Regurgitation

CKD is frequently associated with severe mitral regurgitation (MR).[90] Beyond traditional risk factors, such as diabetes and hypertension, MR results in progressive renal dysfunction by stoke volume reduction and pulmonary hypertension. Invasive surgery in individuals with severe MR and advanced CKD has a high mortality rate.[91] The MitraClip has been proven to be an effective alternative for patients with functional as well as degenerative MR with prohibitive risk for open heart surgery.[92,93] The MitraClip avoids cardio-pulmonary bypass, contrast, or other nephrotoxins and hence is preferable over open heart surgery in patients with CKD. Patients with advanced CKD have relatively lower survival despite percutaneous mitral valve repair.[94–96] There have been multiple studies that demonstrate improvement in renal function after successful MitraClip intervention and occurs in nearly one-third of the cases.[90,94,96–98] A large study of 483 patients demonstrated marked improvement in renal function in CKD stage 4/5 patients after MR reduction to ≤2+ at 1 year.[94] The mechanism behind renal function improvement is probably due to increasing stroke volume and systemic vascular resistance. A similar trend has been seen after transcatheter tricuspid valve repair for severe tricuspid regurgitation.[99] It is unclear which subset of patients will benefit from early intervention with the MitraClip. AKI after MitraClip carries a poor prognosis and the incidence is around 20%.[100,101] Advanced age, euroscore,

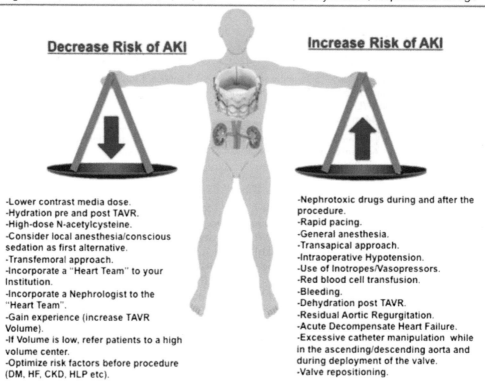

Predisposing Factors for Acute Kidney Injury in TAVR

Age, CKD, PVD, HF, DM, CVA, AF, HLP   Anemia, Dehydration, Nephrotoxic Drugs

Decrease Risk of AKI

-Lower contrast media dose.
-Hydration pre and post TAVR.
-High-dose N-acetylcysteine.
-Consider local anesthesia/conscious sedation as first alternative.
-Transfemoral approach.
-Incorporate a "Heart Team" to your Institution.
-Incorporate a Nephrologist to the "Heart Team".
-Gain experience (increase TAVR Volume).
-If Volume is low, refer patients to a high volume center.
-Optimize risk factors before procedure (DM, HF, CKD, HLP etc).

Increase Risk of AKI

-Nephrotoxic drugs during and after the procedure.
-Rapid pacing.
-General anesthesia.
-Transapical approach.
-Intraoperative Hypotension.
-Use of Inotropes/Vasopressors.
-Red blood cell transfusion.
-Bleeding.
-Dehydration post TAVR.
-Residual Aortic Regurgitation.
-Acute Decompensate Heart Failure.
-Excessive catheter manipulation while in the ascending/descending aorta and during deployment of the valve.
-Valve repositioning.

Fig. 2. Predisposing factors for post-TAVR AKI and potential prevention strategies[108] permission acquired. (*From* Villablanca PA, Ramakrishna H. The Renal Frontier in TAVR. *Journal of cardiothoracic and vascular anesthesia.* 2017;31(3):800-803; with permission.)

preexisting CKD, serum levels of N-terminal pro-B-type natriuretic peptide, hemoglobin A_{1c}, and C-reactive protein are independent predictors of AKI after MitraClip.[100,101] Euvolemia and avoiding nephrotoxins before MitraClip are critical.

Mitral Annular Calcification

MAC is characterized by fibrous, degenerative calcification, and is a common finding in patients with advanced CKD.[7] Functional mitral stenosis or mixed mitral valve disease are common sequalae of MAC. These patients are often poor candidates for invasive cardiac surgery and the use of transcatheter mitral valve replacement (TMVR) seems to be positive. Conduction defects, paravalvular regurgitation, aortic root injury, and LVOT obstruction are complications associated with TMVR.[102] LVOT obstruction is a cataclysmic and unpredictable complication of TMVR. LVOT obstruction is an independent predictor of 1-month (hazard ratio = 3.16; 95% CI, 1.19–8.36) and 1-year mortality (hazard ratio =

3.56; 95% CI, 1.81–7.01). Individuals with severe MAC are at a high risk of LVOT obstruction with rates as high as 54%. This is because of mitral stenosis, small left ventricular cavity, and intact anterior mitral leaflet. The degree of obstruction is influenced by the aortomitral angle and the implantation depth of the device.[103] A neo-LVOT area of less than 1.7 cm^2 is a strong predictor of LVOT obstruction (area under the curve = 0.98, sensitivity = 96.2%, and specificity = 92.3%).[103] Prophylactic alcohol septal ablation or laceration of the anterior mitral leaflet before balloon-expandable device implantation can be considered if the neo-LVOT area is of less than 1.7 cm^2. From an imaging perspective, no standardized protocols are currently available for severe MAC. It is important to assess the mitral annulus dimension; however, this measurement can be challenging in cases of severe calcification or caseous MAC. From a procedural perspective, to decrease embolization of the valve in severe MAC the

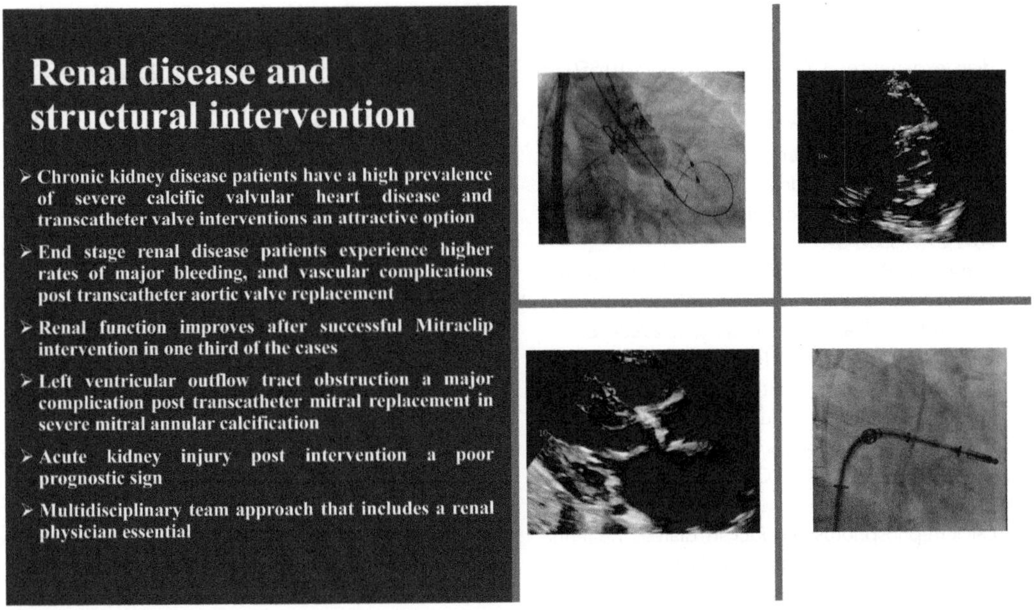

Fig. 3. Renal disease and structural intervention central illustration.

balloon-expandable device should be deployed in tapered orientation and subsequently postdilated within the left ventricle. Mitral valve disease with MAC is linked with high 1-year mortality (odds ratio = 5.44; 95% CI, 3.49–8.49) after TMVR when compared with patients with no MAC.[104] For TMVR, the MAC Global Registry reported 1-month and 1-year all-cause mortality after TMVR of 25% and 53.7%, respectively.[105] The high rates of LVOT obstruction in the registry could be due to heterogenous definition and unreliable assessment of neo-LVOT area on imaging. Preoperative comprehensive evaluation of neo-LVOT area is crucial, preferably multiphase and in particular early systolic,[106] and further studies need to investigate the role of the anterior mitral valve leaflet in preventing LVOT obstruction (LAMPOON) in patients with severe MAC.[107]

SUMMARY AND FUTURE DIRECTIONS

Transcatheter valve interventions have revolutionized the management of severe VHD. The outcomes of patients with CKD after transcatheter valve interventions are worse compared with patients with non-CKD patients. AKI after transcatheter valve interventions are a poor prognostic factor and stringent protocols and teamwork are needed to prevent this complication (Fig. 3). Given the increasing referral base it might be worth considering inclusion of frailty score, comorbidity burden scores, PARTNER TAVI score, or FRANCE 2 TAVI score in the preoperative evaluation of patients undergoing structural intervention on routine basis. Future studies are needed to assess the longevity of devices, quality of life after intervention in this cohort, and furthermore assess the impact of the mode of renal replacement (hemodialysis versus peritoneal dialysis) and outcomes of structural intervention. In addition, it would be interesting to see the impact of CKD/ESRD on valve deterioration, and appropriate timing and impact of valve intervention in patients with CKD to prevent dialysis.

REFERENCES

1. Samad Z, Sivak JA, Phelan M, et al. Prevalence and outcomes of left-sided valvular heart disease associated with chronic kidney disease. J Am Heart Assoc 2017;6(10) [pii:e006044].
2. Wang AY, Wang M, Woo J, et al. Cardiac valve calcification as an important predictor for all-cause mortality and cardiovascular mortality in long-term peritoneal dialysis patients: a prospective study. J Am Soc Nephrol 2003;14(1): 159–68.
3. Sinning JM, Ghanem A, Steinhauser H, et al. Renal function as predictor of mortality in patients after percutaneous transcatheter aortic valve implantation. JACC Cardiovasc Interv 2010;3(11):1141–9.
4. Rodes-Cabau J, Webb JG, Cheung A, et al. Transcatheter aortic valve implantation for the treatment of severe symptomatic aortic stenosis in

patients at very high or prohibitive surgical risk: acute and late outcomes of the multicenter Canadian experience. J Am Coll Cardiol 2010;55(11): 1080–90.

5. Wessely M, Rau S, Lange P, et al. Chronic kidney disease is not associated with a higher risk for mortality or acute kidney injury in transcatheter aortic valve implantation. Nephrol Dial Transplant 2012;27(9):3502–8.

6. Rattazzi M, Bertacco E, Del Vecchio A, et al. Aortic valve calcification in chronic kidney disease. Nephrol Dial Transplant 2013;28(12):2968–76.

7. Ix JH, Shlipak MG, Katz R, et al. Kidney function and aortic valve and mitral annular calcification in the Multi-Ethnic Study of Atherosclerosis (MESA). Am J Kidney Dis 2007;50(3):412–20.

8. Levin NW, Hoenich NA. Consequences of hyperphosphatemia and elevated levels of the calcium-phosphorus product in dialysis patients. Curr Opin Nephrol Hypertens 2001;10(5):563–8.

9. Merjanian R, Budoff M, Adler S, et al. Coronary artery, aortic wall, and valvular calcification in nondialyzed individuals with type 2 diabetes and renal disease. Kidney Int 2003;64(1):263–71.

10. Saran R, Robinson B, Abbott KC, et al. US renal data system 2017 annual data report: epidemiology of kidney disease in the United States. Am J Kidney Dis 2018;71(3 Suppl 1):A7.

11. Perkovic V, Hunt D, Griffin SV, et al. Accelerated progression of calcific aortic stenosis in dialysis patients. Nephron Clin Pract 2003;94(2):e40–5.

12. Maher ER, Young G, Smyth-Walsh B, et al. Aortic and mitral valve calcification in patients with end-stage renal disease. Lancet 1987;2(8564): 875–7.

13. Wang AY, Woo J, Wang M, et al. Association of inflammation and malnutrition with cardiac valve calcification in continuous ambulatory peritoneal dialysis patients. J Am Soc Nephrol 2001;12(9): 1927–36.

14. Yutzey KE, Demer LL, Body SC, et al. Calcific aortic valve disease: a consensus summary from the Alliance of Investigators on Calcific Aortic Valve Disease. Arterioscler Thromb Vasc Biol 2014;34(11):2387–93.

15. de Boer IH, Kestenbaum B, Shoben AB, et al. 25-Hydroxyvitamin D levels inversely associate with risk for developing coronary artery calcification. J Am Soc Nephrol 2009;20(8):1805–12.

16. Hekimian G, Boutten A, Flamant M, et al. Progression of aortic valve stenosis is associated with bone remodelling and secondary hyperparathyroidism in elderly patients—the COFRASA study. Eur Heart J 2013;34(25):1915–22.

17. Drolet MC, Arsenault M, Couet J. Experimental aortic valve stenosis in rabbits. J Am Coll Cardiol 2003;41(7):1211–7.

18. Audet A, Cote N, Couture C, et al. Amyloid substance within stenotic aortic valves promotes mineralization. Histopathology 2012;61(4):610–9.

19. Palaniswamy C, Sekhri A, Aronow WS, et al. Association of warfarin use with valvular and vascular calcification: a review. Clin Cardiol 2011;34(2): 74–81.

20. Han KH, O'Neill WC. Increased peripheral arterial calcification in patients receiving warfarin. J Am Heart Assoc 2016;5(1) [pii:e002665].

21. Koos R, Mahnken AH, Muhlenbruch G, et al. Relation of oral anticoagulation to cardiac valvular and coronary calcium assessed by multislice spiral computed tomography. Am J Cardiol 2005;96(6): 747–9.

22. Ward C. Clinical significance of the bicuspid aortic valve. Heart 2000;83(1):81.

23. Alkhouli M, Alasfar S, Samuels LA. Valvular heart disease and dialysis access: a case of cardiac decompensation after fistula creation. J Vasc Access 2013;14(1):96.

24. Cirit M, Ozkahya M, Cinar CS, et al. Disappearance of mitral and tricuspid regurgitation in haemodialysis patients after ultrafiltration. Nephrol Dial Transplant 1998;13(2):389–92.

25. Massera D, Trivieri MG, Andrews JPM, et al. Disease activity in mitral annular calcification. Circ Cardiovasc Imaging 2019;12(2):e008513.

26. Abramowitz Y, Jilaihawi H, Chakravarty T, et al. Mitral annulus calcification. J Am Coll Cardiol 2015;66(17):1934–41.

27. Abd Alamir M, Radulescu V, Goyfman M, et al. Prevalence and correlates of mitral annular calcification in adults with chronic kidney disease: results from CRIC study. Atherosclerosis 2015; 242(1):117–22.

28. Ozerkan F, Töz H, Ozkahya M, et al. Hypervolemia in dialysis patients—Doppler echocardiography studies. Nephrol Dial Transplant 1998;13(8): 2151–3.

29. Ennezat PV, Marechaux S, Pibarot P. From excessive high-flow, high-gradient to paradoxical low-flow, low-gradient aortic valve stenosis: hemodialysis arteriovenous fistula model. Cardiology 2010;116(1):70–2.

30. Pibarot P, Dumesnil JG. Low-flow, low-gradient aortic stenosis with normal and depressed left ventricular ejection fraction. J Am Coll Cardiol 2012;60(19):1845.

31. Bradley SM, Foag K, Monteagudo K, et al. Use of routinely captured echocardiographic data in the diagnosis of severe aortic stenosis. Heart 2019; 105(2):112.

32. Finegold JA, Manisty CH, Cecaro F, et al. Choosing between velocity-time-integral ratio and peak velocity ratio for calculation of the dimensionless index (or aortic valve area) in serial

follow-up of aortic stenosis. Int J Cardiol 2013; 167(4):1524–31.

33. Rusinaru D, Malaquin D, Marechaux S, et al. Relation of dimensionless index to long-term outcome in aortic stenosis with preserved LVEF. JACC Cardiovasc Imaging 2015;8(7):766–75.

34. Clavel MA, Messika-Zeitoun D, Pibarot P, et al. The complex nature of discordant severe calcified aortic valve disease grading: new insights from combined Doppler echocardiographic and computed tomographic study. J Am Coll Cardiol 2013;62(24):2329–38.

35. Pawade T, Clavel MA, Tribouilloy C, et al. Computed tomography aortic valve calcium scoring in patients with aortic stenosis. Circ Cardiovasc Imaging 2018;11(3):e007146.

36. Wang J, Jagasia DH, Kondapally YR, et al. Comparison of non-contrast cardiovascular magnetic resonance imaging to computed tomography angiography for aortic annular sizing before transcatheter aortic valve replacement. J Invasive Cardiol 2017;29(7):239–45.

37. Harpaz D, Shah P, Bezante G, et al. Transthoracic and transesophageal echocardiographic sizing of the aortic annulus to determine prosthesis size. Am J Cardiol 1993;72(18):1411–7.

38. Straumann E, Meyer B, Misteli M, et al. Aortic and mitral valve disease in patients with end stage renal failure on long-term haemodialysis. Br Heart J 1992;67(3):236.

39. Thourani VH, Sarin EL, Keeling WB, et al. Long-term survival for patients with preoperative renal failure undergoing bioprosthetic or mechanical valve replacement. Ann Thorac Surg 2011;91(4): 1127–34.

40. Horst M, Mehlhorn U, Hoerstrup SP, et al. Cardiac surgery in patients with end-stage renal disease: 10-year experience. Ann Thorac Surg 2000;69(1): 96–101.

41. Brennan JM, Edwards FH, Zhao Y, et al. Long-term survival after aortic valve replacement among high-risk elderly patients in the United States: insights from the Society of Thoracic Surgeons Adult Cardiac Surgery Database, 1991 to 2007. Circulation 2012;126(13):1621–9.

42. Popma JJ, Deeb GM, Yakubov SJ, et al. Transcatheter aortic-valve replacement with a self-expanding valve in low-risk patients. N Engl J Med 2019;380(18):1706–15.

43. Mack MJ, Leon MB, Thourani VH, et al. Transcatheter aortic-valve replacement with a balloon-expandable valve in low-risk patients. N Engl J Med 2019;380(18):1695–705.

44. Leon MB, Smith CR, Mack MJ, et al. Transcatheter or surgical aortic-valve replacement in intermediate-risk patients. N Engl J Med 2016; 374(17):1609–20.

45. Reardon MJ, Van Mieghem NM, Popma JJ, et al. Surgical or transcatheter aortic-valve replacement in intermediate-risk patients. N Engl J Med 2017; 376(14):1321–31.

46. Kodali SK, Williams MR, Smith CR, et al. Two-year outcomes after transcatheter or surgical aortic-valve replacement. N Engl J Med 2012;366(18): 1686–95.

47. Makkar RR, Fontana GP, Jilaihawi H, et al. Transcatheter aortic-valve replacement for inoperable severe aortic stenosis. N Engl J Med 2012; 366(18):1696–704.

48. Vindhyal MR, Ndunda P, Khayyat S, et al. Transcatheter aortic valve replacement and surgical aortic valve replacement outcomes in patients with dialysis: systematic review and meta-analysis. Cardiovasc Revasc Med 2019;20(10):852–7.

49. Amione-Guerra J, Mattathil S, Prasad A. A meta-analysis of clinical outcomes of transcatheter aortic valve replacement in patients with end-stage renal disease. Struct Heart 2018;2(6):548–56.

50. Rattanawong P, Kanitsoraphan C, Kewcharoen J, et al. Chronic kidney disease is associated with increased mortality and procedural complications in transcatheter aortic valve replacement: a systematic review and meta-analysis. Catheter Cardiovasc Interv 2019;94(3):E116–27.

51. Szerlip M, Zajarias A, Vemalapalli S, et al. Transcatheter aortic valve replacement in patients with end-stage renal disease. J Am Coll Cardiol 2019;73(22):2806–15.

52. Allende R, Webb JG, Munoz-Garcia AJ, et al. Advanced chronic kidney disease in patients undergoing transcatheter aortic valve implantation: insights on clinical outcomes and prognostic markers from a large cohort of patients. Eur Heart J 2014;35(38):2685–96.

53. Thourani VH, Forcillo J, Beohar N, et al. Impact of preoperative chronic kidney disease in 2,531 high-risk and inoperable patients undergoing transcatheter aortic valve replacement in the PARTNER trial. Ann Thorac Surg 2016;102(4):1172–80.

54. Szerlip M, Kim RJ, Adeniyi T, et al. The outcomes of transcatheter aortic valve replacement in a cohort of patients with end-stage renal disease. Catheter Cardiovasc Interv 2016;87(7): 1314–21.

55. Hansen JW, Foy A, Yadav P, et al. Death and dialysis after transcatheter aortic valve replacement: an analysis of the STS/ACC TVT Registry. JACC Cardiovasc Interv 2017;10(20):2064–75.

56. Gupta T, Goel K, Kolte D, et al. Association of chronic kidney disease with in-hospital outcomes of transcatheter aortic valve replacement. JACC Cardiovasc Interv 2017;10(20):2050–60.

57. Puri R, Iung B, Cohen DJ, et al. TAVI or No TAVI: identifying patients unlikely to benefit from

transcatheter aortic valve implantation. Eur Heart J 2016;37(28):2217–25.

58. Büttner S, Weiler H, Zöller C, et al. Aortic valve stenosis in a dialysis patient waitlisted for kidney transplantation. Ann Thorac Surg 2016;102(5): e437–8.

59. Orandi BJ, Luo X, Massie AB, et al. Survival benefit with kidney transplants from HLA-Incompatible live donors. N Engl J Med 2016;374(10):940–50.

60. Witberg G, Shamekhi J, Van Mieghem NM, et al. Transcatheter aortic valve replacement outcomes in patients with native vs transplanted kidneys: data from an international multicenter registry. Can J Cardiol 2019;35(9):1114–23.

61. Fox H, Buttner S, Hemmann K, et al. Transcatheter aortic valve implantation improves outcome compared to open-heart surgery in kidney transplant recipients requiring aortic valve replacement. J Cardiol 2013;61(6):423–7.

62. Vemulapalli S, Carroll JD, Mack MJ, et al. Procedural volume and outcomes for transcatheter aortic-valve replacement. N Engl J Med 2019; 380(26):2541–50.

63. Ferro CJ, Chue CD, de Belder MA, et al. Impact of renal function on survival after transcatheter aortic valve implantation (TAVI): an analysis of the UK TAVI registry. Heart 2015;101(7):546.

64. Atsushi O, Masanori Y, Gauthier M, et al. Impact of chronic kidney disease on the outcomes of transcatheter aortic valve implantation: results from the FRANCE 2 registry. EuroIntervention 2015;10(9):e1–9.

65. Thongprayoon C, Cheungpasitporn W, Srivali N, et al. Incidence and risk factors of acute kidney injury following transcatheter aortic valve replacement. Nephrology (Carlton) 2016;21(12):1041–6.

66. Ladia V, Panchal HB, ON TJ, et al. Incidence of renal failure requiring hemodialysis following transcatheter aortic valve replacement. Am J Med Sci 2016;352(3):306–13.

67. Thongprayoon C, Cheungpasitporn W, Srivali N, et al. AKI after transcatheter or surgical aortic valve replacement. J Am Soc Nephrol 2016;27(6): 1854–60.

68. Barbanti M, Gulino S, Capranzano P, et al. Acute kidney injury with the RenalGuard System in patients undergoing transcatheter aortic valve replacement: the PROTECT-TAVI trial (PROphylactic effecT of furosEmide-induCed diuresis with matched isotonic intravenous hydraTion in transcatheter aortic valve implantation). JACC Cardiovasc Interv 2015;8(12):1595–604.

69. Kappetein AP, Head SJ, Genereux P, et al. Updated standardized endpoint definitions for transcatheter aortic valve implantation: the Valve Academic Research Consortium-2 consensus document. Eur Heart J 2012;33(19):2403–18.

70. Najjar M, Salna M, George I. Acute kidney injury after aortic valve replacement: incidence, risk factors and outcomes. Expert Rev Cardiovasc Ther 2015;13(3):301–16.

71. Genereux P, Kodali SK, Green P, et al. Incidence and effect of acute kidney injury after transcatheter aortic valve replacement using the new valve academic research consortium criteria. Am J Cardiol 2013;111(1):100–5.

72. Ram P, Mezue K, Pressman G, et al. Acute kidney injury post-transcatheter aortic valve replacement. Clin Cardiol 2017;40(12):1357–62.

73. Arnold SV, Lei Y, Reynolds MR, et al. Costs of periprocedural complications in patients treated with transcatheter aortic valve replacement: results from the placement of aortic transcatheter valve trial. Circ Cardiovasc Interv 2014;7(6):829–36.

74. Marbach JA, Feder J, Yousef A, et al. Predicting acute kidney injury following transcatheter aortic valve replacement. Clin Invest Med 2017;40(6): E243–51.

75. Wang J, Yu W, Zhou Y, et al. Independent risk factors contributing to acute kidney injury according to updated valve academic research consortium-2 criteria after transcatheter aortic valve implantation: a meta-analysis and meta-regression of 13 studies. J Cardiothorac Vasc Anesth 2017;31(3):816–26.

76. Kolte D, Khera S, Vemulapalli S, et al. Outcomes following urgent/emergent transcatheter aortic valve replacement: insights from the STS/ACC TVT registry. JACC Cardiovasc Interv 2018; 11(12):1175–85.

77. Shishikura D, Kataoka Y, Pisaniello AD, et al. The extent of aortic atherosclerosis predicts the occurrence, severity, and recovery of acute kidney injury after transcatheter aortic valve replacement. Circ Cardiovasc Interv 2018;11(8):e006367.

78. Barbash IM, Ben-Dor I, Dvir D, et al. Incidence and predictors of acute kidney injury after transcatheter aortic valve replacement. Am Heart J 2012; 163(6):1031–6.

79. Bagur R, Webb JG, Nietlispach F, et al. Acute kidney injury following transcatheter aortic valve implantation: predictive factors, prognostic value, and comparison with surgical aortic valve replacement. Eur Heart J 2010;31(7):865–74.

80. Khawaja MZ, Thomas M, Joshi A, et al. The effects of VARC-defined acute kidney injury after transcatheter aortic valve implantation (TAVI) using the Edwards bioprosthesis. EuroIntervention 2012;8(5):563–70.

81. Fefer P, Bogdan A, Grossman Y, et al. Impact of rapid ventricular pacing on outcome after transcatheter aortic valve replacement. J Am Heart Assoc 2018;7(14) [pii:e009038].

82. Elmariah S, Farrell LA, Daher M, et al. Metabolite profiles predict acute kidney injury and mortality

in patients undergoing transcatheter aortic valve replacement. J Am Heart Assoc 2016;5(3): e002712.

83. Zivkovic N, Elbaz-Greener G, Qiu F, et al. Bedside risk score for prediction of acute kidney injury after transcatheter aortic valve replacement. Open heart 2018;5(1):e000777.

84. Brar SS, Aharonian V, Mansukhani P, et al. Haemodynamic-guided fluid administration for the prevention of contrast-induced acute kidney injury: the POSEIDON randomised controlled trial. Lancet 2014;383(9931):1814–23.

85. Yamamoto M, Hayashida K, Mouillet G, et al. Renal function-based contrast dosing predicts acute kidney injury following transcatheter aortic valve implantation. JACC Cardiovasc Interv 2013; 6(5):479–86.

86. Ashworth A, Webb ST. Does the prophylactic administration of N-acetylcysteine prevent acute kidney injury following cardiac surgery? Interact Cardiovasc Thorac Surg 2010;11(3):303–8.

87. Scherner M, Wahlers T. Acute kidney injury after transcatheter aortic valve implantation. J Thorac Dis 2015;7(9):1527–35.

88. Visconti G, Focaccio A, Donahue M, et al. RenalGuard System for the prevention of acute kidney injury in patients undergoing transcatheter aortic valve implantation. EuroIntervention 2016;11(14):e1658–61.

89. He C, Xiao L, Liu J. Safety and efficacy of self-expandable Evolut R vs. balloon-expandable Sapien 3 valves for transcatheter aortic valve implantation: a systematic review and meta-analysis. Exp Ther Med 2019;18(5):3893–904.

90. Kaneko H, Neuss M, Schau T, et al. Interaction between renal function and percutaneous edge-to-edge mitral valve repair using MitraClip. J Cardiol 2017;69(2):476–82.

91. Vassileva CM, Brennan JM, Gammie JS, et al. Mitral procedure selection in patients on dialysis: does mitral repair influence outcomes? J Thorac Cardiovasc Surg 2014;148(1):144–50.e1.

92. Feldman T, Foster E, Glower DD, et al. Percutaneous repair or surgery for mitral regurgitation. N Engl J Med 2011;364(15):1395–406.

93. Obadia J-F, Messika-Zeitoun D, Leurent G, et al. Percutaneous repair or medical treatment for secondary mitral regurgitation. N Engl J Med 2018; 379(24):2297–306.

94. Wang A, Sangli C, Lim S, et al. Evaluation of renal function before and after percutaneous mitral valve repair. Circ Cardiovasc Interv 2015;8(1) [pii: e001349].

95. Estevez-Loureiro R, Settergren M, Pighi M, et al. Effect of advanced chronic kidney disease in clinical and echocardiographic outcomes of patients treated with MitraClip system. Int J Cardiol 2015; 198:75–80.

96. Schueler R, Nickenig G, May AE, et al. Predictors for short-term outcomes of patients undergoing transcatheter mitral valve interventions: analysis of 778 prospective patients from the German TRAMI registry focusing on baseline renal function. EuroIntervention 2016;12(4):508–14.

97. Rassaf T, Balzer J, Rammos C, et al. Influence of percutaneous mitral valve repair using the Mitra-Clip(R) system on renal function in patients with severe mitral regurgitation. Catheter Cardiovasc Interv 2015;85(5):899–903.

98. Kalbacher D, Daubmann A, Tigges E, et al. Impact of pre- and post-procedural renal dysfunction on long-term outcomes in patients undergoing MitraClip implantation: a retrospective analysis from two German high-volume centres. Int J Cardiol 2020;300:87–92.

99. Karam N, Braun D, Mehr M, et al. Impact of transcatheter tricuspid valve repair for severe tricuspid regurgitation on kidney and liver function. JACC Cardiovasc Interv 2019;12(15):1413.

100. Taramasso M, Latib A, Denti P, et al. Acute kidney injury following MitraClip implantation in high risk patients: incidence, predictive factors and prognostic value. Int J Cardiol 2013;169(2):e24–5.

101. Spieker M, Hellhammer K, Katsianos S, et al. Effect of acute kidney injury after percutaneous mitral valve repair on outcome. Am J Cardiol 2018; 122(2):316–22.

102. Tuzcu EM. Trouble after transcatheter mitral valve replacement: anticipate, innovate, refine. JACC Cardiovasc Interv 2019;12(13):1280–2.

103. Yoon SH, Bleiziffer S, Latib A, et al. Predictors of left ventricular outflow tract obstruction after transcatheter mitral valve replacement. JACC Cardiovasc Interv 2019;12(2):182–93.

104. Ribeiro RVP, Yanagawa B, Legare JF, et al. Clinical outcomes of mitral valve intervention in patients with mitral annular calcification: a systematic review and meta-analysis. J Card Surg 2020;35(1):66–74.

105. Guerrero M, Urena M, Himbert D, et al. 1-Year outcomes of transcatheter mitral valve replacement in patients with severe mitral annular calcification. J Am Coll Cardiol 2018;71(17):1841–53.

106. Meduri CU, Reardon MJ, Lim DS, et al. Novel multiphase assessment for predicting left ventricular outflow tract obstruction before transcatheter mitral valve replacement. JACC Cardiovasc Interv 2019;12(23):2402.

107. Khan JM, Babaliaros VC, Greenbaum AB, et al. Anterior leaflet laceration to prevent ventricular outflow tract obstruction during transcatheter mitral valve replacement. J Am Coll Cardiol 2019;73(20):2521–34.

108. Villablanca PA, Ramakrishna H. The renal frontier in TAVR. J Cardiothorac Vasc Anesth 2017;31(3): 800–3.

Pharmacologic Prophylaxis of Contrast-Induced Nephropathy

Anna Toso, MD*, Mario Leoncini, MD, Mauro Maioli, MD, Francesco Bellandi, MD

KEYWORDS

- Contrast-induced nephropathy • Acute kidney injury • Statins • Nicorandil • Trimetazidine

KEY POINTS

- Contrast-induced acute kidney injury (CI-AKI) is a possible complication after angiographic procedures, which exerts a negative prognostic impact in the short- and long-term.
- There is evidence that CI-AKI prevention results in improved clinical outcome.
- No individual drug has received unanimous approval as pharmacologic preventive strategies.
- Short-term statin pretreatment, in association with hydration, is recommended as preventive treatment in the European guidelines for revascularization.
- Shift in paradigm from attention to only CI-AKI to consideration of overall renal damage and its consequences.

PHARMACOLOGIC PROPHYLAXIS OF CONTRAST-INDUCED NEUROPATHY

Our previous review on pharmacologic prophylaxis of contrast-induced acute kidney injury (CI-AKI) for this journal presented the then most studied strategies administered in traditional angiographic procedures.[1] In particular we individuated the characteristics of an ideal drug for CI-AKI prevention, discussed three common agents (statins, N-acetylcysteine, and ascorbic acid), and compared the reported acute benefits on renal functional and clinical benefits over time of these three agents. The findings showed that statins were the most efficacious periprocedural treatment in association with hydration against acute renal damage, leading to better long-term clinical effects.[1] This update, 5 years later, presents an evaluation of the new findings on pharmacologic prevention of CI-AKI dividing statins from all other drugs (Box 1).

STATINS

The most important point underlined in the 2014 review was that "short-term high-dose statin treatment" was an independent protective factor against development of CI-AKI. This fact was based on the results of five randomized controlled trials (RCTs), comparing high-dose statin treatment with placebo or no treatment, published between 2011 and 2014.[2–6] Another crucial issue that emerged was that the benefits in terms of CI-AKI prevention resulted in short- and mid-term favorable impact on clinical outcomes, renal and cardiovascular, but only with statins and not with the other drugs.[1]

WHAT HAS HAPPENED SINCE 2014?

In these intervening years, many authoritative investigators have continued to reconfirm the importance of statins in preventing CI-AKI, especially in patients undergoing cardiologic procedures.[7–10] Recent review of accessible literature evidenced few new randomized trials, all small (minimum of 80 and maximum of 489 patients) and involving a predominance of young men (Table 1).[11–18] High-dose high-potency statins (atorvastatin or rosuvastatin) were administered in all the studies, but they all have different designs, protocols, and patient population characteristics. We note that only half of these trials considered clinical end points (see Table 1).

However, a great number of meta-analyses that included RCTs involving statins were published in

Division of Cardiology, Santo Stefano Hospital, Via Suor Niccolina Infermiera, 20, Prato 59100, Italy
* Corresponding author.
E-mail address: anna.toso@libero.it

Intervent Cardiol Clin 9 (2020) 369–383
https://doi.org/10.1016/j.iccl.2020.02.006

Box 1
Principal drugs administered for CI-AKI prevention
Statins
Other drugs
Allopurinol
α-tocopherol (vitamin E)
Ascorbic acid (vitamin C)
Atrial natriuretic peptide
Bicarbonate/citrate
Calcium channel blockers
Dopamine
Endothelin receptor antagonist
Fenoldopam
Furosemide
Glutathione
L-Arginine
Mannitol
N-Acetylcysteine
Nicorandil
Phosphodiesterase-5 inhibitors
Prednisone
Probucol
Prostacyclin I_2 analogue (iloprost)
Prostaglandin E_1
Theophylline/aminophylline
Trimetazidine

this period (Table 2).[19–39] In all the RCTs in the meta-analyses patients underwent coronary procedures and received short-term statin therapy before contrast medium administration. Statins were demonstrated statistically to be efficacious in preventing CI-AKI in the overall population and various subgroups (diabetes, age groups, gender, contrast volume, type of statin, chronic kidney disease [CKD]). Renal and/or cardiovascular clinical end points were not considered worthy of attention in most of these studies (see Table 2).

TYPE OF STATINS

The statins used in most of the RCTs were atorvastatin or rosuvastatin. The meta-analyses that carried out indirect comparison between atorvastatin and rosuvastatin have not evidenced any remarkable differences between the effects of these two statins even in subgroup analysis.[21,23–25,27,32–34,36,39] To date, there have

been few direct (head-to-head) comparative studies of the two statins. One prospective, observational study by Liu and colleagues[40] compared the effects of rosuvastatin and atorvastatin on CI-AKI in 1078 Chinese patients with CKD undergoing percutaneous coronary intervention (PCI). Periprocedural (2–3 days before and 2–3 days after PCI) treatment with either 10-mg rosuvastatin or 20-mg atorvastatin had similar efficacy for preventing CI-AKI.[40] Two small RCTs involving patients with ST-segment elevation myocardial infarction undergoing primary PCI showed similar results with atorvastatin or rosuvastatin.[41,42] First, the ROSA-CIN study randomized 241 patients with ST-segment elevation myocardial infarction to 80-mg atorvastatin or 40-mg rosuvastatin before PCI.[41] More recently, Firouzi and colleagues[42] randomized 595 patients with ST-segment elevation myocardial infarction for treatment with 80-mg atorvastatin or 40-mg rosuvastatin immediately before primary PCI followed by the same dosages daily up to 48 hours after. Another RCT, the PRATO ACS 2 trial (NCT01870804), focused on 709 patients with non–ST-segment elevation acute coronary syndrome (ACS) treated on hospital admission with atorvastatin (80 mg on-admission followed by 40 mg/d) or rosuvastatin (40 mg on-admission followed by 20 mg/d).

STATINS AND NEPHROPROTECTION

Overall, most available studies and meta-analyses reconfirm the efficacy of statin, in association with routine hydration, as short-term prophylactic strategy against CI-AKI in cardiologic angiographic procedures.[43–46] The current state of knowledge regarding the positive role of statins in CI-AKI prevention is summarized in Box 2. Statins exert numerous metabolic effects, nonlipid mediated (pleiotropic), which derive from the inhibition of mevalonate synthesis and the reduced production of its metabolites (Table 3).[47–50] These effects are rapid (<2 h), which may explain the acute nephroprotective action carried out by the short-term intake of statins before exposure to contrast medium.[49] The nephroprotective effect is well demonstrated in statin-naive patients even after a single dose.[3] Furthermore, the benefits are more marked in high-risk coronary patients (eg, those with ACS or subjected to PCI) in whom the combined action of the multiple pleiotropic effects becomes stronger (eg, antithrombotic, anti-inflammatory, immunomodulatory effects). Therefore, the prevention of CI-AKI, in particular, and kidney

Table 1
Randomized clinical studies with statins after 2014

Author, Ref, Year	Patients (N)	Procedure, Clinical Setting	Mean Age (Males %)	Type and Time of Statin Therapy	CI-AKI Definition Criteria and Results (Treatment vs Control)	Clinical End Points
Shehata and Hamza,[11] 2015	130	Elective CA ± PCI Diabetes and CKD stage 2 or 3	56 ± 5 (62%)	Atorvastatin 80 mg (2 d pre-A) vs placebo	SCr ≥0.5 mg/dL or 25% 72 h 7.7% vs 20%; $P = .05$	NR
Galal et al,[12] 2015	80	CA ± PCI in ACS Diabetes or diabetes and CKD stage 2	56.4 ± 9 (80%)	Atorvastatin 80 mg (12 h pre-A + 40 mg pre-A) vs atorvastatin 10 mg (12 h pre-A + 10 mg pre-A)	Not defined 12.5% vs 17.5%; $P > .05$	NR
Abaci et al,[13] 2015	220	Elective PA or CA ± PCI CKD (eGFR <60 and >30 mL/min)	67.6 ± 8 (68%)	Rosuvastatin 40 mg (24 h pre-A + 20 mg/d 2 d post-A) vs control	SCr ≥0.5 mg/dL or 25% 72 h 5.8% vs 8.5%; $P = .44$	1 y MACE 20% vs 26%; $P = .28$
Bidram et al,[14] 2015	200	Elective CA eGFR >60, without diabetes	60 ± 0.7 (92%)	Atorvastatin 80 mg (12 h pre-A+ 80 mg/d 2 d post-A) vs placebo	SCr ≥0.5 mg/dL or 25% 72 h 1% vs 2%; $P = .77$	NR
Qiao et al,[15] 2015	120	CA ± PCI in ACS Diabetes and CKD stage 2 or 3	61.6 ± 8 (71%)	Atorvastatin 80 mg (1 d pre-A + 80 mg/d 2 d post-A) vs placebo	Peak NGAL: 48 h lower in rosuvastatin ($P = .043$) SCr ≥0.5 mg/dL or 25% 72 h 3% vs 3%; $P > .05$	In-hospital and 30 d MACE No event
Khosravi et al,[16] 2016	220	Elective CA ± PCI Diabetes or CKD (eGFR <60 and >15 mL/min)	63.8 ± 9 (NR)	Atorvastatin 80 mg (2 d pre-A) vs placebo	SCr ≥0.5 mg/dL or 25% 48 h 2.7% vs 10%; $P = .01$	NR
Syed et al,[17] 2017	160	Elective CA ± PCI eGFR >60 and diabetes or hypertension	52.5 ± 8 (62%)	Atorvastatin 80 mg + NAC 1200 mg (3 d pre-A + 2 d post-A) vs NAC 1200 mg	SCr ≥0.5 mg/dL or 25% 48 h 2.5% vs 11.25%; $P = .028$	NR
Fu et al,[18] 2018	489	CA ± PCI in ACS	63 ± 10 (67%)	Atorvastatin 40 mg (1 d pre-A + 3 d post-A) vs atorvastatin 10 mg (1 d pre-A + 3 d post-A)	SCr ≥25% 72 h 6.7% vs 15.1%; $P = .003$ Cystatin C ≥10% 24 h 36.4% vs 18.5%; $P < .001$	In-hospital MACE 2% vs 2%; $P = .47$

Abbreviations: ACS, acute coronary syndrome; CA, coronary angiography; CKD, chronic kidney disease; eGFR, estimated glomerular filtration rate (mL/min/m²); MACE, major adverse cardiovascular events; NAC, N-acetylcysteine; NGAL, neutrophil gelatinase-associated lipocalin; NR, data not reported; PA, peripheral angiography; PCI, percutaneous coronary intervention; post-A, after angiography; pre-A, before angiography; SCr, serum creatinine (mg/dL).

Table 2
Meta-analyses of RCTs with statins

Author, Ref, Year	Number of Trials (Number of Patients)	Clinical Setting	Years of Publication	Statin Dose (Duration of Treatment)	Subgroups Evaluation	CI-AKI (Treatment vs Control)	Clinical Outcomes
Singh et al,[19] 2014	9 (5143)	CA-PCI	2008–2014	High and moderate (short-term)	CKD, NAC use, contrast agent, statin type, diabetes	RR, 0.47 (95% CI, 0.34–0.64; P < .00001)	NR
Mao et al,[20] 2014	6 (1481)	CA-PCI	2008–2013	High and moderate (short-term)	RCT, RC, PC	OR, 0.46 (95% CI, 0.27–0.79; P = .005)	NR
Xie et al,[21] 2014	17 (6323)	CA-PCI	2008–2014	High and low (short-term)	Statin type and dose	OR, 0.50 (95% CI, 0.35–0.71; P < .0001)	30-d mortality
Barbieri et al,[22] 2014	8 (4734)	CA-PCI	2008–2014	High, moderate, and low (short-term)	Statin dose	OR, 0.50 (95% CI, 0.38–0.66; P < .001)	NR
Gandhi et al,[23] 2014	15 (6532) (atorvastatin only)	CA-PCI	2008–2013	High, moderate, and low (short, mid-term, and chronic)	Statin type, statin-naive, ACS, hemodialysis, CKD, diabetes, CHF, contrast volume	RR, 0.59 (95% CI, 0.44–0.80; P = .0005)	NR
Giacoppo et al,[24] 2014	8 (4984)	CA-PCI	2008–2014	High and low (short-term)	CKD, statin type, NAC use, hydration	RR, 0.54 (95% CI, 0.38–0.78; P < .00)	NR
Ukaigwe et al,[25] 2014	12 (5564)	CA-PCI	2008–2014	High and moderate (short-term)	Diabetes, CKD, statin type, NAC use, geography	OR, 0.43 (95% CI, 0.33–0.55; P = .001)	NR
Lee et al,[26] 2014	13 (5825)	CA-PCI	2008–2014	High, moderate, and low (short-term)	ACS, CKD, age, contrast agent, NAC use	RR, 0.45 (95% CI, 0.35–0.57; P < .001)	NR
Liu et al,[27] 2015	5 (5143)	CA-PCI	2008–2014	High, moderate, and low (short-term)	CI-AKI definition, CKD, NAC use, diabetes, statin type	OR, 0.47 (95% CI, 0.37–0.60; P < .0001)	All-cause death
Yang et al,[28] 2015	5 (4045) (rosuvastatin only)	CA-PCI	2012–2015	High and moderate (short-term)	CKD	OR, 0.49 (95% CI, 0.37–0.66; P < .001)	Short-term MACE
Wu et al,[29] 2015	14 (5689) (atorvastatin only)	CA-PCI	2009–2013	High, moderate, and low (short- and mid-term)	PCI	OR, 0.41 (95% CI, 0.29–0.56; P < .001)	NR

Study	No. (Patients)	Procedure	Years	Risk Category	Adjustments	Effect Estimate	MACE
Cheungpasitporn et al,[30] 2015	13 (5803)	CA-PCI–PCeI-PA	2008–2014	High, moderate, and low (short-term)	NR	RR, 0.49 (95% CI, 0.37–0.66; P < .001)	NR
Marenzi et al,[31] 2015	9 (5212)	CA-PCI	2008–2014	High and low (short-term)	ACS	RR, 0.50 (95% CI, 0.39–0.64; P < .001)	NR
Thompson et al,[32] 2016	18 (7161)	CA-PCI-PCeI	2008–2014	High and low (short-term)	ACS, statin type and pretreatment duration, contrast hydration, contrast volume and agent, CKD, geography, NAC use	RR, 0.52 (95% CI, 0.40–0.67; P < .00001)	NR
Wang et al,[33] 2016	14 (6033)	CA-PCI	2008–2014	High, moderate, and low (short-term)	ACS, CKD, age, statin type, NAC use	OR, 0.46 (95% CI, 0.36–0.69; P < .001)	NR
Li et al,[34] 2016	21 (7746)	CA-PCI	2008–2015	High, moderate, and low (short-term, chronic)	Statin type and dose, statin-naive, CI-AKI definition, NAC use, contrast agent	RR, 0.57 (95% CI, 0.47–0.78; P < .00001)	NR
Liang et al,[35] 2017	15 (2673) (rosuvastatin only)	CA-PCI	2012–2016	High, moderate, and low (short-term)	CKD, diabetes, ACS, contrast volume	RR, 0.45 (95% CI, 0.35–0.58; P < .001)	NR
Liu et al,[36] 2018	9 (2210) (atorvastatin only)	CA-PCI	2012–2016	High (short-term)	Time to CI-AKI, CKD, NAC use, diabetes, statin type	OR, 0.46 (95% CI, 0.27–0.79; P < .0004)	NR
Zhang et al,[37] 2018	5 (4057) (rosuvastatin only)	CA-PCI	2013–2014	High and moderate (short-term)	CKD, diabetes	OR, 0.53 (95% CI, 0.40–0.71; P < .0001)	NR
Sun et al,[38] 2019	11 (2752) (atorvastatin only)	CA-PCI	2008–2017	High (short-term)	Statin dose	OR, 0.46 (95% CI, 0.35–0.62; P < .00001)	NR
Zhou et al,[39] 2019	21 (6385)	CA-PCI	2013–2014	High, moderate, and low (short-term)	Statin type and dose	OR, 0.46 (95% CI, 0.37–0.56; P < .0001)	NR

Abbreviations: ACS, acute coronary syndrome; CA, coronary angiography; CHF, congestive heart failure; CI, confidence interval; CKD, chronic kidney disease; MACE, major adverse cardiovascular events; NAC, N-acetylcysteine; NR, data not reported; OR, odds ratio; PA, peripheral angiography; PCeI, percutaneous cerebral artery intervention; PCI, percutaneous coronary intervention; RR, relative risk (95% confidence intervals are reported in parentheses).

Box 2
Efficacy of statins for CI-AKI prevention

Confirmed evidence

- Dose-dependent
- Rapid action
- Independent of LDL reduction
- Noninterference with routine hydration
- Beneficial with all types and volumes of contrast-medium
- Beneficial for all racial populations, but lower dosages in Asian patients
- Beneficial in patients with diabetes
- Beneficial in patients with CKD (eGFR >30 mL/min)
- More efficacious in patients with high CRP levels, ACS, those undergoing PCI procedures

Uncertainties

- Efficacy in severe CKD (eGFR <30 mL/min)
- Efficacy in elderly patients (≥75 years)
- Efficacy in noncardiologic diagnostic/ therapeutic procedures requiring contrast medium

Abbreviations: CRP, C-reactive protein; eGFR, estimated glomerular filtration rate; LDL, low-density lipoprotein.

damage in general is of the utmost importance in patients who undergo diagnostic and therapeutic procedures.

STATINS AND CONTRAST-INDUCED ACUTE KIDNEY INJURY: CURRENT INTERNATIONAL GUIDELINES

The favorable results obtained with the administration of statins have led to the modification of the 2014 and 2018 European guidelines for the prevention of AKI in patients undergoing myocardial revascularization.[51,52] The 2010 international cardiologic guidelines included statins in the term "optimal medical therapy" for patients with CKD (class I) undergoing diagnostic or therapeutic procedures with contrast medium without specifying their short-term prophylactic role in association with hydration strategies.[53] Since 2014 European revascularization guidelines have recommended periprocedural administration of short-term high-dose high-potency statins in statin-naive patients with moderate-to-severe CKD (class IIa) and emphasize the lack of evidence for recommendation of any other pharmacologic strategy.[51,52] This same strategy is recommended by the 2019 European guidelines on dyslipidemia management as short pretreatment or loading (on the background of chronic therapy) for the prevention of CI-AKI (class IIa) in all patients, either stable coronary artery disease or ACS, regardless of renal function.[54] We note that, instead, the US guidelines on myocardial revascularization are still those of 2011 and do not refer to statins as AKI-preventive strategy (Table 4).[52,54–59] Furthermore, in Europe radiologists still do not emphasize any particular therapy for CI-AKI prevention other than routine hydration (see

Table 3
Pathophysiologic mechanisms involved in renal benefits of statins

Statins (HMG-CoA Reductase Inhibitors)	Effects	Time Lapse	Mechanism of Action	Renal Effects
Via reduction of mevalonate metabolites	Pleiotropic mechanisms (non-LDL mediated)	<2 h	Increased NO bioavailability Antioxidant Antiapoptotic Antithrombotic Anti-inflammatory Immunomodulation Antiproliferative Matrix metalloproteinase downregulation Inhibition of tubular protein reuptake	Vasodilation Reduced peritubular and glomerular inflammation Reduced fibrosis Improved hemorheology Improved microcirculation Reduced oxidative stress Albuminuria
Via reduction of cholesterol biosynthesis	LDL-mediated	24–48 h	Lipid reduction	Additional atheroprotective effects

Abbreviations: HMG-CoA, 3-hydroxy-3-methylglutaryl-CoA; LDL, low-density lipoprotein; NO, nitric oxide.

Table 4
Guideline recommendations for pharmacologic preventive measure against CI-AKI

Recommendation	Class of Recommendation	LOE	Guideline
High-dose statins (pretreatment in statin-naive patients with CKD stage 3b and 4)	IIa	A	2018 ESC/EACTS for myocardial revascularization[51]
High-dose statin (routine pretreatment or loading on a background of chronic therapy) before ACS or elective PCI	IIa	B	2019 ESC/EAS for the management of dyslipidemias[52]
Pharmacologic prophylaxis (with statins or other drugs)	Not recommended	A	2018 ESUR on contrast agents[53]
Statins in CKD patients	Not recommended		2012 KDIGO for AKI[54]
Pharmacologic agents	Not specified		2013 NICE for AKI[55]
Pharmacologic agents	Not specified		2011 ACC/AHA/SCAI for PCI[56]
Pharmacologic agents	Not recommended		2012 CAR for prevention of contrast-induced nephropathy[57]

Abbreviations: ACC, American College of Cardiology; AHA, American Heart Association; CAR, Canadian Association Radiology; EACTS, European Association for Cardio-Thoracic Surgery; EAS, European Atherosclerosis Society; ESC, European Society of Cardiology; ESUR, European Society of Urogenital Radiology; KDIGO, Kidney Disease Improving Global Outcomes; LOE, level of evidence; NICE, National Institute for Health and Clinical Excellence; SCAI, Society for Cardiovascular Angiography and Interventions.

Table 4).[55] In fact, to date few reports have been published regarding the use of short-term pharmacologic treatments other than routine hydration in the course of radiologic procedures.[60,61]

OTHER DRUGS

As with statins, in the last 5 years, few RCTs have evaluated the efficacy of other drugs as preventive agents against CI-AKI. Two molecules in particular have attracted attention: nicorandil and trimetazidine. The RCTs and meta-analyses dealing with these drugs are listed in Table 5.[62–81] Both drugs resulted in encouraging findings when administered before elective angiographic procedures in cardiac patients, including those with CKD. However, again, we note the lack of information on post-procedure clinical events.

COMPARISON OF DIFFERENT DRUGS: NETWORK META-ANALYSES

In the last 2 years, six extensive network meta-analyses have been published with the aim of comparing the various preventive strategies, prevalently pharmacologic, used to date.[82–87] The salient data are presented in Table 6. Statins have statistically high ranking for CI-AKI prevention in four of the six meta-analyses. Again, only three of the six studies report data about clinical outcome. When reported this information is

derived from a limited number of the studies included in the respective meta-analysis.[84,85,87]

PHARMACOLOGIC PROPHYLAXIS IN NONCORONARY ANGIOGRAPHIC PROCEDURES

Despite the wide dissemination of the transcatheter aortic valve implantation procedure in recent years, and the increasing awareness of the high incidence of AKI after this complex procedure, it is surprising that no clinical studies are available to date regarding the use of drugs for prophylactic purposes. There are instead numerous reports on the role of different types of hydration or the use of devices (eg, RenalGuard, PLC Medical Systems, Milford, MA) (discussed elsewhere in this issue).

CLINICAL OUTCOME: NEW PARADIGM

In recent years the increasing importance of clinical outcome, beyond renal damage alone, in patients undergoing procedures that use contrast media has been evidenced by the PRESERVE study.[88] This is the first trial to present clinical outcome (a composite of death, the need for dialysis, or a persistent increase in the serum creatinine level of at least 50% from baseline at 90 days after the procedure) as the primary end point, with contrast-associated AKI as secondary end point. Prevention of AKI after

Table 5
Recent studies with nicorandil and trimetazidine

RCTs / Author, Ref, y	Patients (N)	Procedure, Clinical Setting	Mean age (Males %)	Nicorandil Dose and Time of Drug Therapy	CI-AKI Results (Treatment vs Control)	Clinical End Points
Ko et al,[62] 2013	149	Elective CA ± PCI CKD eGFR ≤60 mL/min	70 ± 9.9 (69.8%)	12 mg (IV) (30 min Pre-A) vs control	6.8% vs 6.6%; P = .794	4.1% vs 2.6%; P = .974
Nawa et al,[63] 2015	213	Elective PCI CKD cystatin C >0.95 mg/L in males >0.87 mg/dL in females	70.2 ± 8 (80.2%)	0.096 mg/mL at 0.1 mL/kg/h (IV) (4 h pre-A + 24 h post-A) vs control	2% vs 10.7%; P < .02	NR
Fan et al,[64] 2016	240	Elective CA ± PCI CKD eGFR ≤60 mL/min	66.7 ± 6.35 (76.2%)	30 mg/d (OS) (2 d pre-A + 3 d post-A) vs placebo	6.67% vs 17.5%; P = .017	30-d MACE 4.16% vs 5.83%; P = .767
Iranirad et al,[65] 2017	128	Elective PCI At least 2 CI-AKI risk factors	59.5 ± 12.1 (61.7%)	10 mg (OS) (30 min pre-A + 10 mg/d 3 d post-A) vs control	4.7% vs 21.9%; P = .008	NR
Zhang X et al,[66] 2019	300	Elective CA ± PCI CKD eGFR ≤60 and >30 mL/min	67.2 ± 6.8 (77%)	30 mg/d (OS) (1 d pre-A + 2 d post-A) vs control	3.3% vs 10.7%; P < .05	14-d MACE 3.3% vs 4.0%; P > .05
Zhang P et al,[67] 2019	250	Elective PCI CKD eGFR ≤60 mL/min	67.2 ± 6.9 (72.8%)	30 mg/d (OS) (1 d pre-A + 3 d post-A) vs control	1.6% vs 9.6%; P = .011	In-hospital MACE 4.0% vs 4.8%; P > .05
Fan et al,[68] 2019	252	Elective CA ± PCI CKD eGFR ≤60 mL/min	64 ± 17.2 (57%)	60 mg/d (OS) (2 d pre-A + 2 d post-A) vs control	6.3% vs 15.2%; P = .022	1-y MACE 18% vs 28.8%; P = .032
Zeng et al,[69] 2019	330	Elective CA ± PCI	66.6 ± 7.12 (66%)	30 mg/d (IV) vs 15 mg/d (IV) vs placebo (2 d pre-A + 2 d post-A)	30 mg/d vs placebo: 5.4% vs 14.3%; P = .02; 30 mg/d vs 15 mg/d: 5.4% vs 10.3%; P > .05; 15 mg/d vs placebo: 10.3% vs 14.3%; P > .05	14-d MACE 30 mg/d = 1.8% 15 mg/d = 2.7% placebo = 4.5%; P > .05 (for all comparisons)

Meta-Analyses / Author, Ref, y	Number of Trials (Number of Patients)	Procedure, Clinical Setting	Mean Age (Males %)	Drug Therapy	CI-AKI Results (Treatment vs Control)	Clinical End Points
Wang et al,[70] 2018	4 (730)	Elective CA + PCI CKD	66.7 ± 9 (71.9%)	IV or OS	OR, 0.33 (95% CI, 0.22–0.61; P < .001)	NR
Li et al,[71] 2018	4 (730)	Elective CA + PCI CKD	66.7 ± 9 (71.9%)	IV or OS	RR, 0.36 (95% CI, 0.19–0.74; P = .0001)	NR
Ma et al,[72] 2018	4 (709)	Elective CA ± PCI	66.6 ± 7.8 (72.4%)	IV or OS	RR, 0.37 (95% CI, 0.19–0.74; P = .005)	MACE RR, 0.89 (95% CI, 0.35–2.3; P = .23)

	Author, Ref, y	Patients (N)	Procedure, Clinical Setting	Mean Age (Males %)	Dose and Time of Drug Therapy	CI-AKI Results (Treatment vs Control)	Clinical End Points
	Zhan B et al,[73] 2018	5 (805)	Elective CA ± PCI At least 2 CI-AKI risk factors	65.2 ± 8.7 (70.6%)	IV or OS	RR, 0.37 (95% CI, 0.22–0.61; P = .001	NR
Trimetazidine							
RCTs	Shehata,[74] 2014	100	Elective CA ± PCI Diabetes and CKD stage 2 or 3	58.5 ± 5.5 (68%)	70 mg TMZ + NAC (2 d pre-A + 1 d post-A) vs NAC	12% vs 28%; P < .05	In-hospital events (dialysis, acute heart failure) P > .05
	Liu et al,[75] 2015	132	Elective CA ± PCI CKD stage 2 or 3	58.7 ± 11 (56.8%)	60 mg (2 d pre-A + 1 d post-A) vs control	8% vs 20%; P = .034	1-y MACE 9.6% vs 22.8%; P = .043
	Ye et al,[76] 2017	106	Elective CA ± PCI Diabetes and CKD stage 2 or 3	64.2 ± 8.5 (59.4%)	60 mg (2 d pre-A + 1 d post-A) vs control	9.2% vs 16.7%; P = .043	MACE 7.4% vs 18.5%; P < .05
	Chen et al,[77] 2018	150	Elective CA ± PCI CKD eGFR ≤60 mL/min	62.6 ± 8.5 (55.3%)	60 mg TMZ + CoQ10 (2 d pre-A + 3 d post-A) vs placebo	6.7% vs 21.3%; P = .01	30-d MACE 6.7% vs 8.1%; P = .754
	Mirhosseni et al,[78] 2019	100	Elective CA CKD eGFR ≤60 and >30 mL/min	66.1 ± 6.3 (44%)	70 mg (2 d pre-A + 1 d post-A) vs control	8% vs 20%; P > .05	NR
Observational study	Lian et al,[79] 2019	2154	Elective CA ± PCI	63.4 ± 10.7 (75.2%)	60 mg/d (1 d pre-A until discharge)	9.1% vs 9.2%; P = .947 OR, 0.70 (95% CI, 0.46–1.08; P = .104)	In-hospital MACE 1.89% vs 1.66%; P = .106

	Author, Ref, y	Number of Trials (Number of Patients)	Procedure, Clinical Setting	Mean Age (Males %)	Drug Therapy	CI-AKI Results (Treatment vs Control)	Clinical End Points
Meta-Analyses	Nadkarni et al,[80] 2015	3 RCT (582)	Elective CA ± PCI	58.5 ± 9 (75.8%)	From 60 mg to 70 mg/d (from 2 d pre-A to 3 or 4 d post-A)	5%, 2% vs 16.8%; P < .01 RD, -0.11 (95% CI, -0.16 to -0.06; P < .01)	NR
	Ye et al,[81] 2017	6 RCT (764)	Elective CA ± PCI	60.6 ± 8.4 (NR)	From 60 mg to 70 mg/d (from 2 d pre-A to 3 or 4 d post-A)	OR, 0.27 (95% CI, 0.16–0.46; P < .001)	NR

Abbreviations: CA, coronary angiography; CI, confidence intervals; CoQ10, coenzyme Q10; eGFR, estimated glomerular filtration rate (mL/min/m²); IV, intravenous; MACE, major ative risk; TMZ, trimetazidine.

Table 6
Comparative or network meta-analyses

Author, Ref, Year	Number of Trials (Number of Patients)	Years of Publication	Clinical Setting	Treatment Agents	Reference Strategy	CI-AKI Definition Criteria	Top Ranked Strategies for CI-AKI Prevention (95% CI)	Clinical Outcomes[a]
Su et al,[82] 2017	150 (31,631)	Up to 2016	CA-PCI-CT-PG	11	Saline hydration	SCr ≥0.5 mg/dL or 25% to 48–72 h	HDS: OR, 0.37 (0.16–0.64) HDS + NAC: OR, 0.31 (0.14–0.60)	NA
Giacoppo et al,[83] 2017	124 (28,240)	Up to 2016	CA-PCI	10 (not only drugs)	Saline hydration	SCr ≥0.5 mg/dL or 25% to 48–72 h	S: OR, 0.42 (0.26–0.67) X: OR, 0.32 (0.17–0.57) NAC + NaHCO$_3$: OR, 0.50 (0.33–0.76) NAC: OR, 0.66 (0.47–0.90) NaHCO$_3$: OR, 0.66 (0.47–0.90)	NA
Navarese et al,[84] 2017	147 (33,465)	Up to 2016	CA-PCI	18 (not only drugs)	Saline hydration	SCr ≥0.5 mg/dL or 25% to 48–72 h	PGE$_1$: OR, 0.26 (0.08–0.62) TMZ: OR, 0.26 (0.09–0.59) S: OR, 0.36 (0.21–0.59)	Dialysis, MI, heart failure, mortality
Ma et al,[85] 2018	107 (21,450)	1999–2016	CA-PCI	11	Saline hydration	SCr ≥0.5 mg/dL or 25% to 72 h	PGE$_1$: RR, 0.37 (0.18–0.76) S + NAC: RR, 0.39 (0.21–0.70) BNP: RR, 0.46 (0.30–0.70) S: RR, 0.57 (0.39–0.83) Vitamins: RR, 0.66 (0.45–0.97) NAC + SB: RR, 0.60 (0.39–0.90) NAC: RR, 0.84 (0.17–0.98)	Dialysis, in-hospital and 30-d MACCE, all-cause mortality
Ahmed et al,[86] 2018	200 (42,273)	Up to 2017	CA-PCI-PA-CT-EVAR	44 (not only drugs)	Saline hydration	SCr ≥0.5 mg/dL or 25% to 5 d	PGE$_1$: OR, 0.26 (0.08–0.62) AL: OR, 0.26 (0.08–0.62)	NA
Sharp et al,[87] 2019	48 (14,709)	1999–2018	CA-PCI (only CKD)	7	Saline hydration	SCr ≥0.5 mg/dL or 25% to 48 h	NAC: OR, 077 (0.65–0.91)	Dialysis, MACE, death

Abbreviations: AL, allopurinol; BNP, brain natriuretic peptide; CA, coronary angiography; CI, confidence interval; CT, computed tomography; EVAR, endovascular aneurysm repair; HDS, high-dose statins; MACCE, major adverse cardiac and cerebrovascular events (unstable angina, MI, repeat PCI, heart failure, stroke, all-cause death); MACE, major adverse cardiac events; MI, myocardial infarction; NA, data not reported; NAC, N-acetylcysteine; OR, odds ratio; PA, peripheral angiography; PG, pyelography; PGE$_1$, prostaglandin E$_1$; RR, relative risk; S, statin; SCr, serum creatinine; TMZ, trimetazidine; X, xanthine.

[a] Data derived from a lower number of studies.

angiography procedures is crucial in the attempt to avoid worsening of short- and long-term clinical prognosis.[89] Therefore, in any clinical setting (coronary, peripheral, valvular diagnostic, and/or therapeutic angiographic procedures) one must protect the patient's kidney by combining personalized hydration with personalized optimal medical therapy. The higher the preprocedural risk profile, the greater the work necessary to rebalance all the modifiable parameters that contribute to acute kidney damage.[90–92] Statins represent an effective pharmacologic agent that can be used, also short-term, thanks to their multiple pleiotropic effects, which influence many vulnerable targets. Thus, until now, only statins have been shown to exercise kidney (and cardiac) protection with proven beneficial short- and long-term clinical impact.

DISCLOSURE

The authors have nothing to disclose.

REFERENCES

1. Toso A, Leoncini M, Maioli M, et al. Pharmacologic prophylaxis for contrast-induced acute kidney injury. Interv Cardiol Clin 2014;3:405–19.
2. Patti G, Ricottini E, Nusca A, et al. Short-term, high-dose atorvastatin pretreatment to prevent contrast-induced nephropathy in patients with acute coronary syndromes undergoing percutaneous coronary intervention (from the ARMYDA-CIN [atorvastatin for reduction of myocardial damage during angioplasty–contrast-induced nephropathy] trial. Am J Cardiol 2011;108:1–7.
3. Li W, Fu X, Wang Y, et al. Beneficial effects of high-dose atorvastatin pretreatment on renal function in patients with acute ST-segment elevation myocardial infarction undergoing emergency percutaneous coronary intervention. Cardiology 2012;122: 195–202.
4. Quintavalle C, Fiore D, De Micco F, et al. Impact of a high loading dose of atorvastatin on contrast-induced acute kidney injury. Circulation 2012;126: 3008–16.
5. Han Y, Zhu G, Han L, et al. Short-term rosuvastatin therapy for prevention of contrast-induced acute kidney injury in patients with diabetes and chronic kidney disease. J Am Coll Cardiol 2014;63:62–70.
6. Leoncini M, Toso A, Maioli M, et al. Early high-dose rosuvastatin for contrast-induced nephropathy prevention in acute coronary syndrome: results from the PRATO-ACS Study (protective effect of rosuvastatin and antiplatelet therapy on contrast-induced acute kidney injury and myocardial

damage in patients with acute coronary syndrome). J Am Coll Cardiol 2014;63:71–9.
7. Ball T, McCullough PA. Statins for the prevention of contrast-induced acute kidney injury. Nephron Clin Pract 2014;127:165–71.
8. Briguori C, Napolitano G, Condorelli G. Statins and contrast-induced acute kidney injury. Coron Artery Dis 2014;25:550–1.
9. McCullough PA, Choi JP, Feghali GA, et al. Contrast-Induced acute kidney injury. J Am Coll Cardiol 2016;68:1465–73.
10. Mehran R, Dangas GD, Weisbord SD. Contrast-associated acute kidney injury. N Engl J Med 2019;380:2146–55.
11. Shehata M, Hamza M. Impact of high loading dose of atorvastatin in diabetic patients with renal dysfunction undergoing elective percutaneous coronary intervention: a randomized controlled trial. Cardiovasc Ther 2015;33:35–41.
12. Galal H, Nammas W, Samir A. Impact of high dose versus low dose atorvastatin on contrast induced nephropathy in diabetic patients with acute coronary syndrome undergoing early percutaneous coronary intervention. Egypt Heart J 2015;67: 329–36.
13. Abaci O, Arat Ozkan A, Kocas C, et al. Impact of rosuvastatin on contrast-induced acute kidney injury in patients at high risk for nephropathy undergoing elective angiography. Am J Cardiol 2015;115:867–71.
14. Bidram P, Roghani F, Sanei H, et al. Atorvastatin and prevention of contrast induced nephropathy following coronary angiography. J Res Med Sci 2015;20:1–6.
15. Qiao B, Deng J, Li Y, et al. Rosuvastatin attenuated contrast-induced nephropathy in diabetes patients with renal dysfunction. Int J Clin Exp Med 2015;8: 2342–9.
16. Khosravi A, Dolatkhah M, Hashemi HS, et al. Preventive effect of atorvastatin (80 mg) on contrast-induced nephropathy after angiography in high-risk patients: double-blind randomized clinical trial. Nephrourol Mon 2016;8(3):e29574.
17. Syed MH, Khandelwal PN, Thawani VR, et al. Efficacy of atorvastatin in prevention of contrast-induced nephropathy in high-risk patients undergoing angiography: a double-blind randomized controlled trial. J Pharmacol Pharmacother 2017; 8:50–3.
18. Fu N, Liang M, Yang S. High loading dose of atorvastatin for the prevention of serum creatinine and cystatin C-based contrast-induced nephropathy following percutaneous coronary intervention. Angiology 2018;69:692–9.
19. Singh N, Lee JZ, Huang JJ, et al. Benefit of statin pretreatment in prevention of contrast-induced nephropathy in different adult patient population:

systematic review and meta-analysis. Open Heart 2014;1:e000127.

20. Mao S, Huang S. Statins use and the risk of acute kidney injury: a meta-analysis. Ren Fail 2014;36: 651–7.

21. Xie H, Ye Y, Shan G, et al. Effect of statins in preventing contrast-induced nephropathy: an updated meta-analysis. Coron Artery Dis 2014;25:565–74.

22. Barbieri L, Verdoia M, Schaffer A, et al. The role of statins in the prevention of contrast induced nephropathy: a meta-analysis of 8 randomized trials. J Thromb Thrombolysis 2014;38:493–502.

23. Gandhi S, Mosleh W, Abdel-Qadir H, et al. Statins and contrast-induced acute kidney injury with coronary angiography. Am J Med 2014; 127:987–1000.

24. Giacoppo D, Capodanno D, Capranzano P, et al. Meta-analysis of randomized controlled trials of preprocedural statin administration for reducing contrast-induced acute kidney injury in patients undergoing coronary catheterization. Am J Cardiol 2014;114:541–8.

25. Ukaigwe A, Karmacharya P, Mahmood M, et al. Meta-analysis on efficacy of statins for prevention of contrast-induced acute kidney injury in patients undergoing coronary angiography. Am J Cardiol 2014;114:1295–302.

26. Lee JM, Park J, Jeon KH, et al. Efficacy of short-term high-dose statin pretreatment in prevention of contrast-induced acute kidney injury: updated study-level meta-analysis of 13 randomized controlled trials. PLoS One 2014;9:e111397.

27. Liu YH, Liu Y, Duan CY, et al. Statins for the prevention of contrast-induced nephropathy after coronary angiography/percutaneous interventions: a meta-analysis of randomized controlled trials. J Cardiovasc Pharmacol Ther 2015;20:181–92.

28. Yang Y, Wu YX, Hu YZ. Rosuvastatin treatment for preventing contrast-induced acute kidney injury after cardiac catheterization: a meta-analysis of randomized controlled trials. Medicine (Baltimore) 2015;94:e1226.

29. Wu H, Li D, Fang M, et al. Meta-analysis of short-term high versus low doses of atorvastatin preventing contrast-induced acute kidney injury in patients undergoing coronary angiography/percutaneous coronary intervention. J Clin Pharmacol 2015;55: 123–31.

30. Cheungpasitporn W, Thongprayoon C, Kittanamongkolchai W, et al. Periprocedural effects of statins on the incidence of contrast-induced acute kidney injury: a systematic review and meta-analysis of randomized controlled trials. Ren Fail 2015;37:664–71.

31. Marenzi G, Cosentino N, Werba JP, et al. A meta-analysis of randomized controlled trials on statins for the prevention of contrast-induced acute kidney injury in patients with and without acute coronary syndromes. Int J Cardiol 2015;183:47–53.

32. Thompson K, Razi R, Lee MS, et al. Statin use prior to angiography for the prevention of contrast-induced acute kidney injury: a meta-analysis of 19 randomised trials. EuroIntervention 2016;12: 366–74.

33. Wang N, Qian P, Yan TD, et al. Periprocedural effects of statins on the incidence of contrast-induced acute kidney injury: a systematic review and trial sequential analysis. Int J Cardiol 2016; 2016:143–52.

34. Li H, Wang C, Liu C, et al. Efficacy of short-term statin treatment for the prevention of contrast-induced acute kidney injury in patients undergoing coronary angiography/percutaneous coronary intervention: a meta-analysis of 21 randomized controlled trials. Am J Cardiovasc Drugs 2016;16:201–19.

35. Liang M, Yang S, Fu N. Efficacy of short-term moderate or high-dose rosuvastatin in preventing contrast-induced nephropathy: a meta-analysis of 15 randomized controlled trials. Medicine (Baltimore) 2017;96:e7384.

36. Liu LY, Liu Y, Wu MY, et al. Efficacy of atorvastatin on the prevention of contrast-induced acute kidney injury: a meta-analysis. Drug Des Devel Ther 2018; 12:437–44.

37. Zhang J, Guo Y, Jin Q, et al. Meta-analysis of rosuvastatin efficacy in prevention of contrast-induced acute kidney injury. Drug Des Devel Ther 2018;12: 3685–90.

38. Sun YY, Liu LY, Sun T, et al. Prophylactic atorvastatin prior to intra-arterial administration of iodinated contrast media for prevention of contrast-induced acute kidney injury: a meta-analysis of randomized trial data. Clin Nephrol 2019;92:123–30.

39. Zhou X, Dai J, Xu X, et al. Comparative efficacy of statins for prevention of contrast-induced acute kidney injury in patients with chronic kidney disease: a network meta-analysis. Angiology 2019;70: 305–16.

40. Liu Y, Liu YH, Tan N, et al. Comparison of the efficacy of rosuvastatin versus atorvastatin in preventing contrast induced nephropathy in patient with chronic kidney disease undergoing percutaneous coronary intervention. PLoS One 2014;9:e111124.

41. Kaya A, Kurt M, Tanboga IH, et al. Rosuvastatin versus atorvastatin to prevent contrast induced nephropathy in patients undergoing primary percutaneous coronary intervention (ROSA-CIN trial). Acta Cardiol 2013;68:488–94.

42. Firouzi A, Kazem Moussavi A, Mohebbi A, et al. Comparison between rosuvastatin and atorvastatin for the prevention of contrast-induced nephropathy in patients with STEMI undergoing primary percutaneous coronary intervention. J Cardiovasc Thorac Res 2018;10:149–52.

43. Tropeano F, Leoncini M, Toso A, et al. Impact of rosuvastatin in contrast-induced acute kidney injury in the elderly: post hoc analysis of the PRATO-ACS trial. J Cardiovasc Pharmacol Ther 2016;21:159–66.

44. Rear R, Bell RM, Hausenloy DJ. Contrast-induced nephropathy following angiography and cardiac interventions. Heart 2016;102:638–48.

45. Verdoodt A, Honore PM, Jacobs R, et al. Do statins induce or protect from acute kidney injury and chronic kidney disease: an update review in 2018. J Transl Int Med 2018;6:21–5.

46. Bangalore S. Statins for prevention of contrast-associated acute kidney injury: is the debate a moot point? Cardiovasc Revasc Med 2019;20:632–3.

47. Davignon J. Beneficial cardiovascular pleiotropic effects of statins. Circulation 2004;109(23 Suppl 1):III39–43.

48. Agarwal R. Effects of statins on renal function. Am J Cardiol 2006;97:748–55.

49. Corsini A, Ferri N, Cortellaro M. Are pleiotropic effects of statins real? Vasc Health Risk Manag 2007;3:611–3.

50. Toso A, Leoncini M, De Servi S. Statins and myocardial infarction: from secondary 'prevention' to early 'treatment'. J Cardiovasc Med 2019;20:220–2.

51. Windecker S, Kolh P, Alfonso F, et al. 2014 ESC/EACTS guidelines on myocardial revascularization: the Task Force on Myocardial Revascularization of the European Society of Cardiology (ESC) and the European Association for Cardio-Thoracic Surgery (EACTS) developed with the special contribution of the European Association of Percutaneous Cardiovascular Interventions (EAPCI). Eur Heart J 2014;35:2541–619.

52. Neumann FJ, Sousa-Uva M, Ahlsson A, et al, ESC Scientific Document Group. 2018 ESC/EACTS guidelines on myocardial revascularization. Eur Heart J 2019;40:87–165.

53. Wijns W, Kolh P, Danchin N, et al. Task force on myocardial revascularization of the European Society of Cardiology (ESC) and the European Association for Cardio-Thoracic Surgery (EACTS); European Association for Percutaneous Cardiovascular Interventions (EAPCI), guidelines on myocardial revascularization. Eur Heart J 2010;31:2501–55.

54. Mach F, Baigent C, Catapano AL, et al, ESC Scientific Document Group. 2019 ESC/EAS guidelines for the management of dyslipidaemias: lipid modification to reduce cardiovascular risk. Eur Heart J 2020;41:111–88.

55. van der Molen AJ, Reimer P, Dekkers IA, et al. Post-contrast acute kidney injury. Part 2: risk stratification, role of hydration and other prophylactic measures, patients taking metformin and chronic dialysis patients: recommendations for updated ESUR Contrast Medium Safety Committee guidelines. Eur Radiol 2018;28:2856–69.

56. Kidney Disease: Improving Global Outcomes (KDIGO) Acute Kidney Injury Work Group. KDIGO clinical practice guideline for acute kidney injury. Kidney Int Suppl 2012;2:1–138.

57. National Institute for Health and Care Excellence. Acute kidney injury: prevention, detection and management of acute kidney injury up to the point of renal replacement therapy: NICE clinical guideline 169. London: NICE; 2013. Available at: http://www.nice.org.uk/nicemedia/live/14258/65056/65056.pdf. Accessed December 18, 2013.

58. Guideline for Percutaneous Coronary Intervention. A report of the American College of Cardiology Foundation/American Heart Association Task Force on practice guidelines and the Society for Cardiovascular Angiography and Interventions 2011 ACCF/AHA/SCAI. J Am Coll Cardiol 2011;58:e44–122.

59. Owen RJ, Hiremath S, Myers A, et al. Canadian Association of Radiologists consensus guidelines for the prevention of contrast-induced nephropathy: update 2012. Can Assoc Radiol J 2014;65:96–105.

60. Sanei H, Hajian-Nejad A, Sajjadieh-Kajouei A, et al. Short term high dose atorvastatin for the prevention of contrast-induced nephropathy in patients undergoing computed tomography angiography. ARYA Atheroscler 2014;10:252–8.

61. Palli E, Makris D, Papanikolaou J, et al. The impact of N-acetylcysteine and ascorbic acid in contrast-induced nephropathy in critical care patients: an open-label randomized controlled study. Crit Care 2017;21:269.

62. Ko YG, Lee BK, Kang WC, et al. Preventive effect of pretreatment with intravenous nicorandil on contrast-induced nephropathy in patients with renal dysfunction undergoing coronary angiography (PRINCIPLE Study). Yonsei Med J 2013;54:957–64.

63. Nawa T, Nishigaki K, Kinomura Y, et al. Continuous intravenous infusion of nicorandil for 4 hours before and 24 hours after percutaneous coronary intervention protects against contrast-induced nephropathy in patients with poor renal function. Int J Cardiol 2015;195:228–34.

64. Fan Y, Wei Q, Cai J, et al. Preventive effect of oral nicorandil on contrast-induced nephropathy in patients with renal insufficiency undergoing elective cardiac catheterization. Heart Vessels 2016;31:1776–82.

65. Iranirad L, Hejazi SF, Sadeghi MS, et al. Efficacy of nicorandil treatment for prevention of contrast-induced nephropathy in high-risk patients undergoing cardiac catheterization: a prospective randomized controlled trial. Cardiol J 2017;24:502–7.

66. Zhang X, Yang S, Zhang P, et al. Efficacy of nicorandil on the prevention of contrast-induced nephropathy in patients with coronary heart disease undergoing percutaneous coronary intervention. Coron Artery Dis 2019. https://doi.org/10.1097/MCA.0000000000000826.

67. Zhang P, Li WY, Yang SC, et al. Preventive effects of nicorandil against contrast-induced nephropathy in patients with moderate renal insufficiency undergoing percutaneous coronary intervention. Angiology 2019;71:183–8.

68. Fan Z, Li Y, Ji H, et al. Efficacy of oral nicorandil to prevent contrast-induced nephropathy in patients with chronic renal dysfunction undergoing an elective coronary procedure. Kidney Blood Press Res 2019;44:1372–82.

69. Zeng Z, Fu X, Zhang X, et al. Comparison of double-dose vs. usual dose of nicorandil for the prevention of contrast-induced nephropathy after cardiac catheterization. Int Urol Nephrol 2019;51:1999–2004.

70. Wang X, Geng J, Zhu H, et al. Renoprotective effect of nicorandil in patients undergoing percutaneous coronary intervention: a meta-analysis of 4 randomized controlled trials. Oncotarget 2018;9:11837–45.

71. Li S, Wang L, Liu Y, et al. Preventive effect of nicorandil on contrast-induced nephropathy: a meta-analysis of randomised controlled trials. Intern Med J 2018;48:957–63.

72. Ma X, Li X, Jiao Z, et al. Nicorandil for the prevention of contrast-induced nephropathy: a meta-analysis of randomized controlled trials. Cardiovasc Ther 2018;36:e12316.

73. Zhan B, Huang X, Jiang L, et al. Effect of nicorandil administration on preventing contrast-induced nephropathy: a meta-analysis. Angiology 2018;69:568–73.

74. Shehata M. Impact of trimetazidine on incidence of myocardial injury and contrast-induced nephropathy in diabetic patients with renal dysfunction undergoing elective percutaneous coronary intervention. Am J Cardiol 2014;114:389–94.

75. Liu W, Ming Q, Shen J, et al. Trimetazidine prevention of contrast-induced nephropathy in coronary angiography. Am J Med Sci 2015;350:398–402.

76. Ye Z, Lu H, Su Q, et al. Effect of trimetazidine on preventing contrast-induced nephropathy in diabetic patients with renal insufficiency. Oncotarget 2017;8:102521–30.

77. Chen F, Liu F, Lu J, et al. Coenzyme Q10 combined with trimetazidine in the prevention of contrast-induced nephropathy in patients with coronary heart disease complicated with renal dysfunction undergoing elective cardiac catheterization: a randomized control study and in vivo study. Eur J Med Res 2018;23:23.

78. Mirhosseni A, Farahani B, Gandomi-Mohammadabadi A, et al. Preventive effect of trimetazidine on contrast-induced acute kidney injury in CKD patients based on urinary neutrophil Gelatinase-associated Lipocalin (uNGAL): a randomized clinical trial. Iran J Kidney Dis 2019;13:191–7.

79. Lian X, He W, Zhan H, et al. The effect of trimetazidine on preventing contrast-induced nephropathy after cardiac catheterization. Int Urol Nephrol 2019. https://doi.org/10.1007/s11255-019-02308-w.

80. Nadkarni GN, Konstantinidis I, Patel A, et al. Trimetazidine decreases risk of contrast-induced nephropathy in patients with chronic kidney disease: a meta-analysis of randomized controlled trials. J Cardiovasc Pharmacol Ther 2015;20:539–46.

81. Ye Z, Lu H, Su Q, et al. Clinical effect of trimetazidine on prevention of contrast-induced nephropathy in patients with renal insufficiency: an updated systematic review and meta-analysis. Medicine (Baltimore) 2017;96:e6059.

82. Su X, Xie X, Liu L, et al. Comparative effectiveness of 12 treatment strategies for preventing contrast-induced acute kidney injury: a systematic review and bayesian network meta-analysis. Am J Kidney Dis 2017;69:69–77.

83. Giacoppo D, Gargiulo G, Buccheri S, et al. Preventive strategies for contrast-induced acute kidney injury in patients undergoing percutaneous coronary procedures: evidence from a hierarchical bayesian network meta-analysis of 124 trials and 28 240 patients. Circ Cardiovasc Interv 2017;10 [pii:e004383].

84. Navarese EP, Gurbel PA, Andreotti F, et al. Prevention of contrast-induced acute kidney injury in patients undergoing cardiovascular procedures-a systematic review and network meta-analysis. PLoS One 2017;12:e0168726.

85. Ma WQ, Zhao Y, Wang Y, et al. Comparative efficacy of pharmacological interventions for contrast-induced nephropathy prevention after coronary angiography: a network meta-analysis from randomized trials. Int Urol Nephrol 2018;50:1085–95.

86. Ahmed K, McVeigh T, Cerneviciute R, et al. Effectiveness of contrast-associated acute kidney injury prevention methods; a systematic review and network meta-analysis. BMC Nephrol 2018;19:323.

87. Sharp AJ, Patel N, Reeves BC, et al. Pharmacological interventions for the prevention of contrast-induced acute kidney injury in high-risk adult patients undergoing coronary angiography: a systematic review and meta-analysis of randomised controlled trials. Open Heart 2019;6:e000864.

88. Weisbord SD, Gallagher M, Jneid H, et al, PRESERVE Trial Group. Outcomes after angiography

with sodium bicarbonate and acetylcysteine. N Engl J Med 2018;378:603–14.

89. Kooiman J, Seth M, Nallamothu BK, et al. Association between acute kidney injury and in-hospital mortality in patients undergoing percutaneous coronary interventions. Circ Cardiovasc Interv 2015;8: e002212.

90. Kellum JA, Bellomo R, Ronco C. Progress in prevention and treatment of acute kidney

injury: moving beyond kidney attack. JAMA 2018;320:437–8.

91. Koyner J, Bakris G. Kidney injury is not prevented by hydration alone. Eur Heart J 2019;40:3179–81.

92. James MT, Har BJ, Tyrrell BD, et al. Clinical decision support to reduce contrast-induced kidney injury during cardiac catheterization: design of a randomized stepped-wedge trial. Can J Cardiol 2019;35:1124–33.

Hydration

Intravenous and Oral: Approaches, Principals, and Differing Regimens: Is It What Goes in or What Comes Out That Is Important?

Richard Solomon, MD

KEYWORDS

- Acute kidney injury • Hydration • Contrast • Diuresis • Intravenous fluid • Urine output

KEY POINTS

- Kidney injury following the administration of contrast occurs; estimates from large databases suggest an incidence of ~5% following intravenous contrast and 5% to 15% following intra-arterial contrast. The term contrast-associated acute kidney injury (CA-AKI) best describes this phenomenon.
- CA-AKI is associated with adverse short-term and long-term events. Whether it is causal is unclear.
- Prevention of CA-AKI is the most important approach as there is no treatment of CA-AKI once it occurs.
- Current guidelines (American College of Radiology, American Heart Association/American College of Cardiology, Society for Cardiovascular Angiography and Interventions) suggests providing adequate hydration and minimizing contrast volume as the most evidence-based approaches to prevention of CA-AKI.
- Inducing a high urine flow rate may be the key to preventing CA-AKI.

INTRODUCTION AND CURRENT GUIDELINES

Acute kidney injury (AKI) following administration of contrast media occurs in up to 5% to 15% of patients undergoing diagnostic and interventional angiography, although the incidence may be higher in certain high-risk subgroups. AKI may also occur following administration of contrast for computed tomography (CT) examinations. Whether the contrast media causes the injury is increasingly controversial and therefore such kidney injury is now referred to as postcontrast AKI or contrast-associated AKI (CA-AKI).[1] This article uses the latter term. Regardless of the role of contrast, when CA-AKI occurs, it is associated with adverse short-term and long-term outcomes.[2] Because there is no treatment of CA-AKI once it occurs, strategies are focused on prevention and include identifying high-risk patients, minimizing the amount of contrast used, and providing intravenous fluids, particularly to high-risk patients.[3,4]

The American Heart Association (AHA) foundation and American College of Cardiology (ACC) issued guidelines in 2011 for prevention and a major recommendation (grade 1A) included that "appropriate preparatory hydration" be used in high-risk patients.[4] The writing group found the evidence insufficient to

Division of Nephrology, Larner College of Medicine, University of Vermont, University of Vermont Medical Center, UHC 2309, 1 South Prospect Street, Burlington, VT 05401, USA
E-mail address: Richard.Solomon@uvmhealth.org

Intervent Cardiol Clin 9 (2020) 385–393
https://doi.org/10.1016/j.iccl.2020.02.009

recommend a specific fluid regime. In 2012, the Kidney Disease: Improving Global Outcomes (KDIGO) Acute Kidney Injury Workgroup upgraded recommendations regarding prevention of CA-AKI.[5] They recommended intravenous volume expansion with either isotonic sodium chloride or sodium bicarbonate solutions, rather than no intravenous volume expansion, in patients at increased risk for CI-AKI (1A). They also recommended not using oral fluids alone in patients at increased risk of CI-AKI (1C).

These recommendations lack specificity and leave decisions about fluid administration to the discretion of the physicians caring for the patients. Since these recommendations were upgraded, 2 important trials have been published. The AMACING (A MAstricht Contrast-Induced Nephropathy Guideline) trial reported that intravenous fluid administration was not superior to no fluid administration at least for low-risk patients with estimated glomerular filtration rate (eGFR) greater than 30 mL/min.[6] This guideline led to a revision of ESUR (European Society of Urogenital Radiology) guidelines suggesting intravenous fluids only in patients with eGFR less than 30 mL/min or where there was first-pass renal exposure to contrast.[7] A subsequent study in patients with eGFR less than 30 mL/min could not confirm the benefit of intravenous fluids, although a trend toward benefit was evident.[8] The PRESERVE (Prevention of Serious Adverse Events Following Angiography) trial found no differences between sodium chloride and sodium bicarbonate on 90-day end points of death, dialysis, or sustained 50% increase in serum creatinine (MAKE-D) as well as no difference in the incidence of CA-AKI.[9] Follow-up analyses of this trial suggested that the risk of MAKE-D (Major adverse kidney events - dialysis) was minimal in patients with CA-AKI (under review, *Journal of the American College of Cardiology* [JACC]), although this has been challenged (under review, JACC). Importantly the updated guidelines and the recent studies, do not address mechanisms that may be involved in the protective effect of fluid administration, leaving many to question the basis of the guidelines.

This article concentrates on what constitutes adequate fluid administration based on the author's understanding of the mechanisms of protection against AKI and evidence from randomized clinical trials. A key theme is that, although the guidelines focus on what to give the patient, it may be that what comes out of the patient (urine) is the critical element.

MECHANISMS OF INJURY (FLUID ADMINISTRATION SHOULD HAVE SOME EFFECT IN ABROGATING THESE MECHANISM)

Contrast nephrotoxicity occurs as a result of multiple mechanisms, including (1) ischemia, primarily caused by intrarenal vasoconstriction; (2) tubule cell toxicity mediated by increased oxidative stress; and (3) slowing of intratubular flow because of the viscosity of the contrast media (See Shweta Bansal and Rahul N. Patel's article, "Pathophysiology of Contrast-Induced Acute Kidney Injury," in this issue). Evidence supporting these mechanisms includes the following: contrast media increase the production of reactive oxygen species (ROS)[10] through mitochondrial damage and endothelin,[11] leading to renal vasoconstriction, particularly in the vasa recti supplying blood to the outer medulla. The renal outer medulla is the most sensitive part of the kidney to ischemia because of its unique vascular anatomy and high metabolic rate.[12] The high oxygen consumption is generated by the active transport of sodium in the S3 segment of the proximal tubule and the ascending limb of Henle. At the same time, there is decreased delivery of oxygen to this area. The vasa recti supplying blood and oxygen follow the loop of Henle, and the close proximity of the descending and ascending vasa recti allows oxygen to diffuse out of the oxygen-rich descending vessels into the oxygen-depleted ascending vessels. The result is that tissue oxygen levels in the medulla are approximately 50% that of the renal cortex (20 mm Hg vs 40 mm Hg).[12] The balance between oxygen delivery and oxygen consumption in this part of the kidney can be upset by contrast media.[13] For example, contrast media with an osmolality greater than serum (low-osmolar contrast media [LOCM]) induce an osmotic diuresis with more sodium delivery to the loop of Henle and therefore more oxygen consumption. In addition, the increased sodium delivery to the macula densa stimulates tubuloglomerular feedback, resulting in afferent arteriolar vasoconstriction and a decrease in vasa recti blood flow. Consumption goes up and oxygen delivery goes down. Contrast media with an osmolality similar to plasma (iso-osmolar contrast media [IOCM]) are considerably more viscous than LOCM and result in slowing of flow in the vasa recti, leading to a decrease in oxygen delivery[14] and a slowing of flow in the renal tubule that could increase contact time between the contrast media and the renal tubule epithelium.

All contrast media (both LOCM and IOCM) are also directly toxic to renal tubule cells. The cells take up the contrast into the cytoplasm where injury to mitochondrial membranes occurs, leading to apoptosis, a common final pathway for most causes of AKI.[15,16] Recently animal data using intravital microscopy have shown that contrast contact time within the proximal tubule is markedly increased in dehydrated rats. This increase in contact time results in contrast being taken up by peritubular macrophages, resulting in the production of inflammatory cytokines and an inflammatory injury to the kidney.[17]

A new animal model uses dehydration and furosemide to increase the incidence of AKI following contrast administration to rats.[18] In summary, ischemia, direct toxicity, and inflammation all can contribute to the reduction in glomerular filtration rate (GFR) that identifies CA-AKI.

ORAL VERSUS INTRAVENOUS FLUID

Four prospective trials randomized patients to a prescribed amount of oral water or 0.9% sodium chloride before and after contrast exposure. These trials included a total of only 399 patients with normal to impaired kidney function undergoing arteriography (coronary in 3 of 4 trials). There were no differences in the incidence of CA-AKI between the oral water and intravenous sodium chloride groups.[19–22] The total amount of oral water given was between 1100 and 2500 mL for the period 6 hours before to 24 hours after contrast exposure. Although the evidence base is limited and many of these patients would be considered low risk, these trials raise the hypothesis that urine output (which is vigorous after a water load) rather than volume expansion (which would be considerably less with oral water compared with intravenous isotonic crystalloid) may be of critical importance. A recent meta-analysis of oral versus intravenous fluid trials came to the same conclusion and in addition found the combination of water and intravenous fluid to be the most effective prophylactic strategy.[23] Regardless of whether water intake alone is sufficient to reduce the incidence of CA-AKI, both water intake and urine output before and after contrast administration must be considered as important confounding variables in assessing the results of any clinical trial.

EVIDENCE OF BENEFICIAL EFFECT OF INTRAVENOUS FLUID ON CONTRAST-ASSOCIATED ACUTE KIDNEY INJURY FROM CLINICAL TRIALS

Eisenberg and colleagues[24] in 1981 first made the observation that AKI was absent in patients who received a lot of intravenous and oral fluid during and after angiography. Since that time, many observational studies have confirmed the original observation. Additional prospective randomized trials have compared different types of fluid administration, including oral versus intravenous,[25,26] hypotonic versus isotonic intravenous fluid,[27] and intravenous sodium chloride versus sodium bicarbonate.[28] However, it is only recently that prospective randomized trials have compared giving any fluid with a no-fluid control group.[29–31] In these initial studies, patients with an ST-elevation myocardial infarction (STEMI) were studied. Because of the imperative to get patients into the catheterization laboratory as quickly as possible, these patients receive little to no preangiography fluid (oral or intravenous). Furthermore, their courses after angiography are often complicated by cardiac dysfunction. They are therefore at high risk for CA-AKI.

Two of the 3 trials randomized a total of 624 patients with STEMI to no fluid or isotonic sodium chloride at 1 mL/kg/h for either 12[30] or 24 hours[29] after angiography. Both found a marked reduction in the incidence of AKI favoring fluid administration, defined as an increase in serum creatinine level of 25% or 44.4 μmol/L over baseline during the following 72 hours. These studies in high-risk patients are to be contrasted with prospective randomized trials in low-risk patients; that is, those undergoing contrast-enhanced CT examinations and elective cardiac angiography. In a study of 138 patients with a baseline eGFR of less than 60 mL/min/1.73 m^2, no difference was found between withholding fluids and giving 250 mL of isotonic sodium bicarbonate.[32] A recent trial (AMACING) that included patients undergoing a contrast-enhanced CT or elective angiography compared no fluid with intravenous isotonic sodium chloride given before and after contrast exposure. Again, there was no difference in the incidence of AKI, which was low (~2%).[6] However, the AMACING trial was underpowered and enrolled only 40% of the expected number. Only 92 patients underwent an intervention. In addition, both trials did not control for oral fluid intake (discussed earlier). Fig. 1 shows the data for interventional procedures in these randomized trials.

Although fluid administration was shown to be superior to no fluid for prevention of AKI in high-risk patients (STEMI), the trials could not address whether giving fluid before angiography was of importance. Furthermore, administration of large amounts of fluid after angiography increases the volume of distribution of creatinine and therefore reduces the rate of increase in serum creatinine level in the setting of a decrease in GFR. The third

Randomized trials of fluid vs no fluid for patients getting interventional procedures

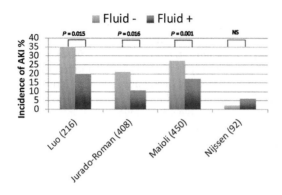

Fig. 1. Prospective randomized trials comparing no fluid administration with intravenous 0.9% sodium chloride. The numbers in parentheses are the numbers of subjects in each study. NS, nonsignificant. (*Data from* Refs.[6,29–31])

trial, by Maioli and colleagues,[31] attempted to address the issue of timing of fluid administration by randomizing patients with STEMI to 1 of 3 groups: no fluid (control group), a preangiography administration of sodium bicarbonate 3 mL/kg/h for 1 hour followed by sodium chloride 1 mL/kg/h for 12 hours (early hydration), or just sodium chloride 1 mL/kg/h for 12 hours following angiography (late hydration). The patients who received preangiography fluid had the lowest incidence of AKI (control 27.3%, early 12.0%, and late 22.7%). However, it was the amount of fluid administered regardless of timing that was critical. Dividing the patients by tertiles of fluid administered, there was a progressive decrease in AKI as more fluid was given (26.7% for the lowest tertile, 17.0% for the middle tertile, and 8.1% for the highest tertile) regardless of when it was given. The take-home message was that the more fluid you give, the better the prophylaxis of AKI, so the volume of administered fluid is more important than timing. As mentioned earlier, this observation might also be confounded by increasing the volume of distribution for creatinine.

If administering a large volume of fluid is beneficial, particularly in high-risk patients, how do clinicians determine how much fluid to give and how to give it safely? There is a risk of volume expanding patients too much, resulting in heart failure and arrhythmias.[33] Several studies have found a higher risk of these adverse events in patients given large amounts of isotonic fluid, and retrospective data analyses have found that higher administered volume was also associated with more AKI.[34] One approach to minimizing the risk of cardiovascular complications is to

adjust fluid administration using cardiac hemodynamic monitoring. The POSEIDON (Prevention of Contrast Renal Injury with Different Hydration Strategies) trial used left ventricular end-diastolic pressure (LVEDP) at the start of coronary angiography to adjust the rate of fluid administration and compared these hemodynamic-guided patients with a control group that received a standard rate of 0.9% sodium chloride.[35] The patients who underwent hemodynamic monitoring had a lower incidence of AKI compared with the controls (6.7% vs 16.3%, $P = .005$), but they also received nearly twice as much fluid (1727 mL vs 812 mL, $P = .0001$). Assessing tertiles of fluid administration, the incidence of AKI was 17% in the lowest, 11% in the middle, and 6% in the highest tertile for volume administration, again supporting the argument that more fluid is protective. A second trial used dynamic changes in central venous pressure (CVP) during angiography to adjust fluid administration rates. The group that had fluid administration guided by CVP again received more fluid (1827 mL vs 1202 mL, $P = .001$), made more urine (1461 mL vs 806 mL, $P = .001$), and had a lower incidence of AKI (15.9% vs 29.5%, $P = .006$).[36] These trials provide further support for the concept that more fluid is better for prevention of AKI.

THE IMPORTANCE OF URINE OUTPUT

The PRINCE (The Prevention of Radiocontrast Induced Nephropathy Clinical Evaluation) trial was an attempt to specifically reduce CA-AKI by increasing urine output through a combination of intravenous fluid, diuretics (furosemide and mannitol), and renal vasodilators (dopamine).[37]

The trial showed that subjects achieving an average urine output greater than 150 mL/h over the first 24 hours after angiography had a reduced incidence of CA-AKI. Furthermore, urine outputs greater than ≈260 mL/h for the first 24 hours were associated with no change in serum creatinine level over the ensuing 48 hours (**Fig. 2**). Based on these results, attempts to increase urine output as a preventive strategy were widely adopted. These trials used mannitol or furosemide to force a diuresis. However, a seminal randomized trial of saline alone or saline plus mannitol or saline plus furosemide showed that the saline-alone group had the lowest incidence of CA-AKI.[38] Three subsequent randomized trials confirmed that adding furosemide to intravenous fluid to force a diuresis increased the incidence of CA-AKI.[25,39,40]

An inherent problem with this strategy was that patients were in negative fluid balance. Furthermore, the doses of furosemide used were high (~1 mg/kg intravenous). Although an increase in urine output might be beneficial, these trials showed that diuresis cannot occur at the expense of hypovolemia. Producing volume depletion, even a small amount, seems to override any potential benefit.

Forced Matched Diuresis

A solution to inducing a diuresis without volume depletion was provided with a device that matched intravenous fluid administration milliliter for milliliter with urine output in real time. The system continually weighs the urine collection bag and uses changes in weight to drive a pump to deliver an equivalent amount of isotonic saline intravenously. Slight volume expansion is initiated with a small intravenous fluid bolus (250 mL of isotonic sodium chloride) followed by a low dose of furosemide (0.25 mg/kg) to increase urine output. Urine output is driven to 300 to 800 mL/h for approximately 6 hours (**Fig. 3**) with no net change in extracellular volume. To date, more than 1000 patients undergoing invasive angiography procedures have been studied, with most of them in randomized prospective trials.[41–45] The results have been consistent and impressive (**Fig. 4**). Few adverse effects on serum electrolyte levels have occurred and all trials have found a significant reduction in the incidence of CA-AKI. Furthermore, the incidence of CA-AKI was inversely related to the amount of urine output[46] despite the similar initial bolus of fluid. With a reduction in the incidence of CA-AKI, there were also benefits in terms of long-term adverse cardiovascular events.[47] A recent trial, REMEDIAL III (Renal Insufficiency After Contrast Media Administration III), compared forced matched diuresis with hemodynamic-guided fluid administration using LVEDP.[48] Forced matched diuresis was superior to hemodynamic-guided fluid administration, both for CA-AKI and long-term adverse events (data presented at 2019 Transcatheter Cardiovascular Therapeutics meeting in San Francisco, CA). The urine output was considerably greater in the forced matched diuresis group. What these studies highlight is that increasing urine output in the absence of volume depletion is protective against CA-AKI.

WHAT IS THE MECHANISM OF BENEFIT?

How does fluid administration or a high urine output interfere with any of the pathophysiologic processes mentioned earlier that contribute to kidney injury from contrast administration? It

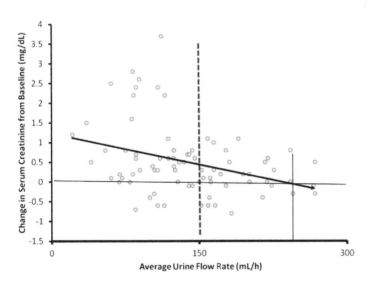

Fig. 2. The relationship between average urine flow rate over 24 hours after angiography and change in serum creatinine level. Adapted from PRINCE study. (*From* Stevens MA, McCullough P, Tobin K et al. A prospective randomized trial of prevention measures in patients at high risk for contrast nephropathy. J Am Coll Cardiol 1999;33:403-411; with permission.)

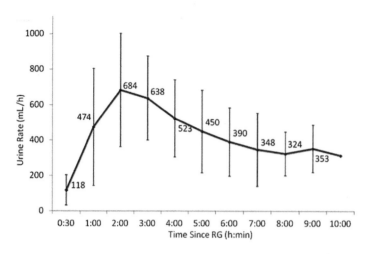

Fig. 3. Trajectory of hourly urine output and intravenous fluid administration achieved with the forced matched hydration protocol. RG, RenalGuard. (*From* Dorval JF, Dixon SR, Zelman RB, Davidson CJ, Rudko R, Resnic FS. Feasibility study of the RenalGuard balanced hydration system: a novel strategy for the prevention of contrast-induced nephropathy in high risk patients. International journal of cardiology 2013;166:482-6; with permission.)

must do so either by improving the balance between oxygen delivery and consumption or diminishing direct cell toxicity and inflammation by reducing contact time between the renal epithelium and the contrast medium.

Intuitively, a reduction in direct renal tubule cell toxicity might be expected from the high urine flow rate. The direct nephrotoxicity of contrast is highly time dependent, beginning within 15 minutes of exposure and increasing over the following hours.[49] The concentration of contrast within the tubule lumen would be reduced by a high urine flow rate. In animal models, giving intravenous fluid before contrast administration also reduces the viscosity of the urine following administration of a variety of contrast media (IOCM and LOCM), supporting a reduction in contrast concentration within the urine.[50] Reducing the concentration of sodium

and chloride in the fluid that reaches the macula densa could also reduce the tubuloglomerular feedback response.[51]

Contrast media induce an increase in ROS as part of the mechanisms producing vasa recti vasoconstriction leading to medullary ischemia. One direct measurement of this effect is that contrast media reduce medullary tissue oxygen levels in animals as assessed by blood oxygen level detection MRI.[13] In contrast, high urine flow rates induced by water drinking increase medullary oxygen levels.[52] A water load (20 mL/kg over 15 minutes) in humans results in an increase in medullary oxygen levels within minutes in normal individuals, although this effect is blunted by prostaglandin inhibition, in elderly subjects, and in patients with diabetes.[52,53] Whether such an effect underlies the benefits of a high urine flow rate in patients exposed to contrast is untested.

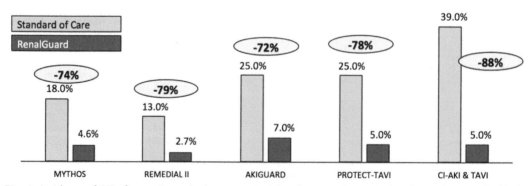

Fig. 4. Incidence of AKI after angiography (coronary, peripheral, transcatheter aortic valve replacement) with the forced matched hydration strategy compared with a control group receiving intravenous isotonic fluid for the same amount of time. AKIGUARD, Acute Kidney Injury Guarding Device; MYTHOS, Induced Diuresis With Matched Hydration Compared to Standard Hydration for Contrast Induced Nephropathy Prevention; PROTECT-TAVI, Prophylactic Effect of Furosemide-induced Diuresis with Matched Isotonic Intravenous Hydration in Transcatheter Aortic Valve Implantation; REMEDIAL, Renal Insufficiency Following Contrast Media Administration Trial; TAVI, transcatheter aortic valve implantation. (*Data from* Refs.[41–45])

Box 1
Recommendations for achieving adequate hydration for patients at risk of acute kidney injury from exposure to contrast media

1. Hold diuretics on the day of contrast exposure (exception: patients with decompensated heart failure or when performing forced matched diuresis).

2. Administer isotonic crystalloid with a goal to correct clinical evidence of decreased renal perfusion (exception: patients in decompensated heart or liver failure).

3. Discontinue pharmacologic agents that predispose to decreased vasa recti perfusion: nonsteroidal antiinflammatory drug (randomized trial [RT]).

4. Change nil-by-mouth orders to allow for drinking of water up to 2 hours before angiography.

5. Induce a vigorous urine flow rate with intravenous fluid and oral water. This rate is most important after contrast exposure but ideally should be started before exposure. The goal is to produce a flow rate greater than 150 mL/h after contrast for at least 4 hours (RT). Thus, at least 150 mL of total fluid (oral and intravenous) needs to be administered per hour.

6. In high-risk patients (including decompensated heart and liver failure), use of a device that matches intravenous fluids to urine output can ensure a large urine output without inducing extracellular volume changes (RT).

These recommendations represent the author's opinion. Randomized trials (RT) support most of these recommendations.

In addition, preventing volume depletion itself may be additionally protective. Volume depletion is a recognized risk factor for all causes of AKI, perhaps because intrarenal vasoconstriction is activated under these conditions. Such vasoconstriction could exacerbate the vasoconstrictive effects of contrast media. Furthermore, intrinsic antioxidant defense mechanisms are impaired in volume-depleted animals.[54] Correcting volume depletion with an initial bolus of isotonic fluid before angiography could help mitigate the damaging effects of ROS generated by contrast media.

SUMMARY

The evidence presented in this article supports the hypothesis that high urine flow rates and the avoidance of hypovolemia are protective against contrast nephrotoxicity and clinical CA-AKI. It is difficult to achieve these high urine flow rates (>300 mL/h) without risking volume depletion unless an automated system is used for matching urine output and intravenous fluid administration in real time. Box 1 lists recommendations appropriate for most settings. Future research is needed to further define the mechanisms by which a high urine flow rate is protective.

DISCLOSURE

Dr R. Solomon is a member of the scientific advisory committee for 3 device companies: Sonogenix, Medi-Beacon, and PLC Med Inc. All are interested in early diagnosis and prevention of AKI. Dr R. Solomon is a subprincipal investigator on National Institutes of Health study IMPROVE AKI: a cluster-randomized trial of team-based coaching interventions to improve acute kidney injury.

REFERENCES

1. Weisbord SD, du Cheryon D. Contrast-associated acute kidney injury is a myth: No. Intensive Care Med 2018;44:107–9.

2. Cho JY, Jeong MH, Hwan Park S, et al. Effect of contrast-induced nephropathy on cardiac outcomes after use of nonionic isosmolar contrast media during coronary procedure. J Cardiol 2010;56: 300–6.

3. Thomsen HS. Guidelines for contrast media from the European Society of Urogenital Radiology. AJR Am J Roentgenol 2003;81:1463–71.

4. Wright RS, Anderson JL, Adams CD, et al. 2011 ACCF/AHA focused update of the guidelines for the management of patients with unstable angina/non-ST-elevation myocardial infarction (updating the 2007 guideline): a report of the American College of Cardiology Foundation/American Heart Association Task Force on Practice Guidelines developed in collaboration with the American College of Emergency Physicians, Society for Cardiovascular Angiography and Interventions, and Society of Thoracic Surgeons. J Am Coll Cardiol 2011;57:1920–59.

5. (KDIGO) AKIWGKDIGO. Clinical practice guideline for acute kidney injury. Kidney Int Suppl 2012;2:1–138.

6. Nijssen EC, Rennenberg RJ, Nelemans PJ, et al. Prophylactic hydration to protect renal function from intravascular iodinated contrast material in patients at high risk of contrast-induced nephropathy (AMACING): a prospective, randomized, phase 3, controlled, open-label, non-inferiority trial. Lancet 2017;389(10076):1312–22.

7. van der Molen AJ, Reimer P, Dekkers IA, et al. Post-contrast acute kidney injury. Part 2: risk stratification, role of hydration and other prophylactic measures, patients taking metformin and chronic dialysis patients: Recommendations for updated ESUR Contrast Medium Safety Committee guidelines. Eur Radiol 2018;28:2856–69.

8. Nijssen EC, Nelemans PJ, Rennenberg RJ, et al. Prophylaxis in high-risk patients with eGFR < 30 mL/min/1.73 m2. Invest Radiol 2019;54:580–8.

9. Weisbord SD, Gallagher M, Jneid H, et al. Outcomes after angiography with sodium bicarbonate and acetylcysteine. N Engl J Med 2018;378(7):603–14.

10. Heyman SN, Rosen S, Khamaisi M, et al. Reactive oxygen species and the pathogenesis of radiocontrast-induced nephropathy. Invest Radiol 2010;45:188–95.

11. Hentschel M, Gildein P, Brandis M, et al. Endothelin (ET-1) is involved in the contrast media induced nephrotoxicity in children with congenital heart disease. Clin Nephrol 1995;43:s12–5.

12. Brezis M, Rosen S. Hypoxia of the renal medulla-its implications for disease. N Engl J Med 1995;332:647–55.

13. Li LP, Franklin T, Du H, et al. Intrarenal oxygenation by blood oxygenation level-dependent MRI in contrast nephropathy model: effect of the viscosity and dose. J Magn Reson Imaging 2012;36:1162–7.

14. Sendeski M, Patzak A, Persson PB. Constriction of the vasa recta, the vessels supplying the area at risk for acute kidney injury, by four different iodinated contrast media, evaluating ionic, nonionic, monomeric and dimeric agents. Invest Radiol 2010;45:453–7.

15. Quintavalle C, Anselmi CV, De Micco F, et al. Neutrophil Gelatinase-associated lipocalin and contrast-induced acute kidney injury. Circ Cardiovasc Interv 2015;8:e002673.

16. Fanning NF, Manning BJ, Buckley J, et al. Iodinated contrast media induce neutrophil apoptosis through a mitochondrial and caspase mediated pathway. Br J Radiol 2002;75:861–73.

17. Lau A, Chung H, Komada T, et al. Renal immune surveillance and dipeptidase-1 contribute to contrast-induced acute kidney injury. J Clin Invest 2018;128:2894–913.

18. Cheng W, Zhao F, Tang CY, et al. Comparison of iohexol and iodixanol induced nephrotoxicity, mitochondrial damage and mitophagy in a new contrast-induced acute kidney injury rat model. Arch Toxicol 2018;92:2245–57.

19. Cho R, Javed N, Traub D, et al. Oral hydration and alkalinization is noninferior to intravenous therapy for prevention of contrast-induced nephropathy in patients with chronic kidney disease. J Interv Cardiol 2010;23:460–6.

20. Kong D, YF H, Ma LL, et al. Comparison of oral and intravenous hydration strategies for the prevention of contrast-induced nephropathy in patients undergoing coronary angiography or angioplasty: a randomized clinical trial. Acta Cardiol 2012;67:565–9.

21. Lawlor D, Moist D, Derose L, et al. Prevention of contrast-induced nephropathy in vascular surgery patients. Ann Vasc Surg 2007;21:593–7.

22. Wrobel W, Sinkiewicz W, Gordon M, et al. Oral versus intravenous hydration and renal function in diabetic patients undergoing percutaneous coronary interventions. Kardiol Pol 2010;68:1015–20.

23. Zhang WD, Zhang JW, Yang BJ, et al. Effectiveness of oral hydration to prevent contrast-induced acute kidney injury in patients undergoing coronary angiography or intervention: a pairwise and network meta-analysis. Coron Artery Dis 2018;29(4):286–93.

24. Eisenberg RL, Bank WO, Hedgock MW. Renal failure after major angiography can be avoided with hydration. Am J Radiol 1981;136:859–61.

25. Dussol B, Morange S, Loundoun A, et al. A randomized trial of saline hydration to prevent contrast nephropathy in chronic renal failure patients. Nephrol Dial Transplant 2006;21:2120–6.

26. Trivedi HS, Moore H, Nasr S, et al. A randomized prospective trial to assess the role of saline hydration on the development of contrast nephrotoxicity. Nephron Clin Pract 2003;93:c29–34.

27. Mueller C, Buerkle G, Buettner H, et al. Prevention of contrast media-associated nephropathy: randomized comparison of 2 hydration regimens in 1620 patients undergoing coronary angiography. Arch Intern Med 2002;162:329–36.

28. Merten G, Burgess WG, Gray LV, et al. Prevention of contrast-induced nephropathy with sodium bicarbonate: a randomized controlled trial. JAMA 2004;291:2328–34.

29. Jurado-Roman A, Hernandez-Hernandez F, Garcia-Tejada J, et al. Role of hydration in contrast-induced nephropathy in patients who underwent primary percutaneous coronary intervention. Am J Cardiol 2015;115:1174–8.

30. Luo Y, Wang X, Ye Z, et al. Remedial hydration reduces the incidence of contrast-induced nephropathy and short-term adverse events in patients with ST-segment elevation myocardial infarction: a single-center, randomized trial. Intern Med 2014;53:2265–72.

31. Maioli M, Toso A, Leoncini M, et al. Effects of hydration in contrast-induced acute kidney injury after primary angioplasty: a randomized, controlled trial. Circ Cardiovasc interventions 2011;4:456–62.

32. Kooiman J, Sijpkens YW, van Buren M, et al. Randomised trial of no hydration vs. sodium bicarbonate hydration in patients with chronic kidney disease undergoing acute computed

tomography-pulmonary angiography. J Thromb Haemost 2014;12:1658–66.

33. Liu Y, Li H, Chen S, et al. Excessively high hydration volume may not be associated with decreased risk of contrast-induced acute kidney injury after percutaneous coronary intervention in patients with renal insufficiency. J Am Heart Assoc 2016;5 [pii: e003171].

34. Bei WJ, Wang K, Li HL, et al. Safe hydration to prevent contrast-induced acute kidney injury and worsening heart failure in patients with renal insufficiency and heart failure undergoing coronary angiography or percutaneous coronary intervention. Int Heart J 2019;60:247–54.

35. Brar S, and the Poseidon investigators. A prospective, randomized trial of sliding-scale hydration for the prevention of contrast nephropathy. presented at TCT (abst) 2012.

36. Qian G, Fu Z, Guo J, et al. Prevention of contrast-induced nephropathy by central venous pressure-guided fluid administration in chronic kidney disease and congestive heart failure patients. JACC Cardiovasc Interv 2016;9:89–96.

37. Stevens MA, McCullough P, Tobin K, et al. A prospective randomized trial of prevention measures in patients at high risk for contrast nephropathy. J Am Coll Cardiol 1999;33:403–11.

38. Solomon R, Werner C, Mann D, et al. Effects of saline, mannitol, and furosemide to prevent acute decreases in renal function induced by radiocontrast agents. N Engl J Med 1994;331:1416–20.

39. Majumdar SR, Kjellstrand CM, Tymchak WJ, et al. Forced euvolemic diuresis with mannitol and furosemide for prevention of contrast-induced nephropathy in patients with CKD undergoing coronary angiography: a randomized controlled trial. Am J Kidney Dis 2009;54:602–9.

40. Weinstein JM, Heyman S, Brezis M. Potential deleterious effect of furosemide in radiocontrast nephropathy. Nephron 1992;62:413–5.

41. Barbanti M, Gulino S, Capranzano P, et al. Acute kidney injury with the RenalGuard system in patients undergoing transcatheter aortic valve replacement: the PROTECT-TAVI Trial (PROphylactic effecT of furosEmide-induCed diuresis with matched isotonic intravenous hydraTion in Transcatheter Aortic Valve Implantation). JACC Cardiovasc Interv 2015;8:1595–604.

42. Briguori C, Visconti G, Focaccio A, et al. Renal insufficiency after contrast media administration trial II (REMEDIAL II): RenalGuard system in high-risk patients for contrast-induced acute kidney injury. Circulation 2011;124:1260–9.

43. Marenzi G, Ferrari C, Marana I, et al. Prevention of contrast nephropathy by furosemide with matched hydration: the MYTHOS (induced diuresis with matched hydration compared to standard hydration for contrast induced nephropathy prevention) trial. JACC Cardiovasc Interv 2012;5:90–7.

44. Usmiani T, Andreis A, Budano C, et al. AKIGUARD (Acute Kidney Injury GUARding Device) trial: in-hospital and one-year outcomes. J Cardiovasc Med 2015;17:530–7.

45. Visconti G, Focaccio A, Donahue M, et al. Renal-Guard System for the prevention of acute kidney injury in patients undergoing transcatheter aortic valve implantation. Eurointervention 2016;11:e1658–61.

46. Briguori C, Visconti G, Donahue M, et al. RenalGuard system in high-risk patients for contrast-induced acute kidney injury. Am Heart J 2016;173:67–76.

47. Putzu A, Boscolo Berto M, Belletti A, et al. Prevention of contrast-induced acute kidney injury by furosemide with matched hydration in patients undergoing interventional procedures: a systematic review and meta-analysis of randomized trials. JACC Cardiovasc Interv 2017;10:355–63.

48. Briguori C, D'Amore C, De Micco F, et al. Renal insufficiency following contrast media administration trial III: Urine flow rate-guided versus left-ventricular end-diastolic pressure-guided hydration in high-risk patients for contrast-induced acute kidney injury. Rationale and design. Catheter Cardiovasc Interv 2019. [Epub ahead of print].

49. Romano G, Briguori C, Quintavalle C, et al. Contrast agents and renal cell apoptosis. Eur Heart J 2008;29:2569–76.

50. Seeliger E, Flemming B, Wronski T, et al. Viscosity of contrast media perturbs renal hemodynamics. J Am Soc Nephrol 2007;18:2912–20.

51. Vallon V. Tubuloglomerular feedback and the control of glomerular filtration rate. News Physiol Sci 2003;18:169–74.

52. Tumkur SM, Vu AT, Li LP, et al. Evaluation of intrarenal oxygenation during water diuresis: a time-resolved study using BOLD MRI. Kidney Int 2006;70:139–43.

53. Prasad PV, Epstein FH. Changes in renal medullary pO2 during water diuresis as evaluated by blood oxygenation level-dependent magnetic resonance imaging: effects of aging and cyclooxygenase inhibition. Kidney Int 1999;55:294–8.

54. Yoshioka Y, Fogo A, Beckman JK. Reduced activity of antioxidant enzymes underlies contrast media-induced renal injury in volume depletion. Kidney Int 1992;41:1008–15.

Device Based Approaches to the Prevention of Contrast-Induced Acute Kidney Injury

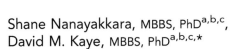

Shane Nanayakkara, MBBS, PhD[a,b,c],
David M. Kaye, MBBS, PhD[a,b,c,*]

KEYWORDS

• Renal failure • Acute kidney injury • Creatinine • Pre-hydration • Contrast media

---

KEY POINTS

- Contrast-induced acute kidney injury occurs in up to 30% of high-risk patients undergoing percutaneous coronary intervention.
- Pharmacologic approaches are of limited benefit; multiple device-based approaches exist to reduce contrast exposure, guide hydration, and provide renal protection.
- Newer technologies also permit low or zero contrast intervention, to significantly reduce the potential of acute kidney injury.
- Early results are promising; however, large randomized controlled trials powered to detect hard clinical end points are required to prove feasibility and benefit of these devices in patients at risk of kidney injury.

INTRODUCTION

Key Mechanisms of Contrast-Induced Acute Kidney Injury

The development of contrast-induced acute kidney injury (CI-AKI) depends on the physiochemical properties of contrast media, specifically the viscosity and osmolality of the contrast used, in combination with the vasoactive and directly cytotoxic effects. This cytotoxicity leads to a prolonged period of vasoconstriction after contrast administration, with a sequence of ischemia to the outer medulla and release of vasoactive mediators that lead to renal dysfunction.[1] Reactive oxygen species are released, increasing oxidative stress.[2] Hypovolemia increases the concentration of contrast media in the tubules, decreasing clearance, and hypotension exacerbates renal hypoperfusion and ischemia.[2] Embolization of atheroemboli from coronary and structural procedures from the femoral approach can also result in renal injury. Consequently, it follows that therapies to target these specific mechanisms may be of most benefit in preventing CI-AKI (**Fig. 1**).

Direct Renal Protection
Remote ischemic conditioning
In view of the dominant theory of renal ischemic injury associated with contrast being related to ischemia and oxidative stress, remote ischemic preconditioning has been hypothesized as a

---

[a] Department of Cardiology, Alfred Hospital, 55 Commercial Road, Melbourne, VIC 3004, Australia; [b] Department of Medicine, Nursing and Health Sciences, Monash University, Wellington Road, Clayton, Melbourne, VIC 3168, Australia; [c] Heart Failure Research Group, Baker Heart and Diabetes Institute, 75 Commercial Road, Melbourne, VIC 3004, Australia
* Corresponding author. Department of Cardiology, Alfred Hospital, 55 Commercial Road, Melbourne, VIC 3004, Australia.
E-mail address: d.kaye@alfred.org.au
Twitter: @DrNanayakkara (S.N.)

Intervent Cardiol Clin 9 (2020) 395–401
https://doi.org/10.1016/j.iccl.2020.02.005
2211-7458/20/© 2020 Elsevier Inc. All rights reserved.

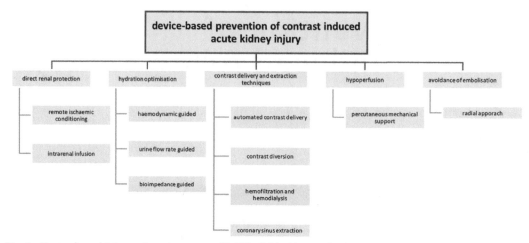

Fig. 1. Device-based interventions to prevent CI-AKI, divided by mechanism.

potential preventative therapy. In a randomized, blinded, sham-controlled study of 100 patients with impaired renal function (estimated glomerular filtration rate of <60 mL/min/1.73 m^2) undergoing coronary angiography, Er and colleagues[3] performed preconditioning using four 5-minute cycles of inflation and deflation to 50 mm Hg greater than the patients systolic blood pressure, beginning immediately before angiography. There was a marked reduction in CI-AKI development (odds ratio [OR], 0.21; 95% confidence interval 0.07–0.57; P = .002). Results were similar in patients with moderate and severe renal dysfunction, although the overall study was relatively small. Postconditioning works on a similar principle, involving sequential alternating coronary balloon 30-second inflation/deflation cycles after percutaneous coronary intervention (PCI). A randomized study of 225 patients undergoing PCI demonstrated a similar significant reduction in CI-AKI (OR, 0.34; 95% confidence interval, 0.16–0.71).[4] Both methods are of interest owing to their relatively inexpensive nature and ease of translation into clinical practice; however, larger studies with longer term follow-up are required to evaluate the true clinical benefit.

Intrarenal infusion

The Benephit catheter (AngioDynamics, Latham, NY) is a bifurcated catheter designed to engage both renal arteries to infuse fenoldopam, a drug hypothesized to increase renal blood flow. Although an early registry of 501 patients demonstrated a lower incidence of CI-AKI than predicted by the Mehran score,[5] the device is not currently clinically available and development seems to have ceased.

HYDRATION OPTIMIZATION

It is well-established that prehydration for those with impaired baseline renal function is beneficial in preventing renal injury, however the optimal rate and volume are unclear. Current guidelines recommend intravascular volume expansion with intravenous administration of normal saline (1–1.5 mL/kg/h) for at least 6 hours before and after contrast exposure. Two primary methods have been used to guide clinicians, based on either the left ventricular end-diastolic pressure (LVEDP) or the urine flow rate. Trials of both studies have shown decreases in CI-AKI, noting that patients randomized to either strategy often receive significantly more fluid than patients randomized to standard care.

Left Ventricular End-Diastolic Pressure–Guided Optimization

One simple metric on which to guide fluid administration is the LVEDP, frequently measured as a part of routine cardiac catheterization. Although frequently performed ad hoc by clinicians, few studies have measured the impact on clinical outcomes using a standardized protocol. The Prevention of Contrast Renal Injury with Different Hydration Strategies (POSEIDON) trial[6] assigned 396 patients to either standard care (weight-based prehydration) or the same together with intravenous fluid rates based on the LVEDP: patients received 5 mL/kg/h if the LVEDP was less than 13 mm Hg, 3 mL/kg/h if the LVEDP was 13 to 18 mm Hg, and 1.5 mL/kg/h if the LVEDP was greater than 18 mm Hg. The mean glomerular filtration rate was 48 mL/min/1.73 m^2. There was a significant decrease in CI-AKI (6.7% in the intervention arm vs 16.4% in the standard care group; $P = .005$). Follow-up out to 6 months showed a persistent benefit on hard clinical outcomes; those treated with the LVEDP-guided method had a significant reduction in the composite end point of death, myocardial infarction, or dialysis (relative risk, 0.32; 95% confidence interval, 0.13–0.79; $P = .008$) with statistically significant reductions in each clinical end point. As expected, the overall volume administered was significantly higher in the intervention group (1711 mL vs 807 mL; $P<.001$), with 3 patients in each group developing pulmonary edema, requiring diuresis and cessation of therapy.

Urine Flow Rate–Guided Optimization

Increasing the urine flow rate through controlled hydration has shown protective effects against the development of CI-AKI. Forced diuresis with frusemide should theoretically result in similar protective effects, although this has not been borne out in trials, perhaps owing to systemic or renal hemodynamic changes exacerbated by the subsequent delivery of contrast.[7]

The RenalGuard (RenalGuard Solutions Inc, Milford, MA) is a closed loop fluid replacement system that uses a standard urinary Foley catheter and intravenous fluid set to automatically replace fluid in real-time. An early study comparing the device to bicarbonate and N-acetylcysteine had shown benefit (OR, 0.47; 95% confidence interval, 0.24–0.92) in patients with an estimated glomerular filtration rate of 30 mL/min/1.73 m^2 or less. Recently, the Renal Insufficiency Following Contrast Media Administration (REMEDIAL III) trial[8] was a 708 patient multicentre randomized controlled trial comparing the role of the urine flow rate–guided optimization with LVEDP-guided hydration. Patients with baseline chronic kidney disease (estimated glomerular filtration rate of ≤45 mL/min/1.73 m^2) and at high risk for the development of CI-AKI (based on either the Mehran[9] or Gurm[10] scores) were included. Hydration volumes were significantly higher in the urine flow rate–guided arm (2700 mL vs 1700 mL). The primary end point, a composite of CI-AKI and/or pulmonary edema, occurred in just more than one-half as many patients in the urine flow rate–guided arm (relative risk, 0.56; 95% confidence interval, 0.39–0.79), primarily driven by CI-AKI. Follow-up to 30 days continued in favor of the urine flow rate–guided arm. Importantly, hypokalemia was significantly more frequent (6.2% vs 2.3%; $P = .013$). Drawbacks to the device include cost and the requirement of a urinary catheter,

both as an additional discomfort and risk to the patient, and also as a potential delay in procedure time and turnover.

Bioimpedance Vector Analysis

Bioimpedance reflects the overall fluid volume (total body water), a measure that is reasonably well-correlated with intravascular volume. Electrodes are placed on the hand and foot, with the patient in a supine position for 5 minutes. A graph comparing resistance and reactance (indexed to height) is then generated with the patient plotted to evaluate fluid status. Maioli and colleagues[11] recently evaluated the role of bioimpedance vector analysis in 1018 patients undergoing coronary angiography. Patients were divided into those with an optimal body fluid level or a low body fluid level based on the initial admission bioimpedance vector analysis measurement; those with a low level (n = 303) were randomized to 1 mL/kg/h or 2 mL/kg/h, with a half rate for all patients with an ejection fraction of less than 40% or clinical signs and symptoms of heart failure. An automated injector was used in all cases. Using the standard definition of CI-AKI (serum creatinine level of ≥0.3 mg/dL within 48 hours), there was a nonstatistically significant decrease in the 2 mL/kg/h arm (4.7% vs 10.8%; $P = .08$), which was significant using the trial's primary end point of an increase in cystatin C of 10% or greater within 24 hours (OR, 0.45; 95% confidence interval, 0.24–0.85; $P = .015$). A subgroup analysis showed a benefit in all patients except those with a left ventricular ejection fraction of less than 40%, although the study was small and perhaps underpowered for subgroup analysis.

Hypoperfusion

Patients with hypotension, cardiogenic shock, or significant left ventricular systolic dysfunction are at risk of AKI in the context of the double hit of ischemia associated with contrast media. High-risk PCI procedures are increasingly being supported with percutaneous mechanical support devices such as the Impella (Abiomed, Danvers, MA). These devices can provide short-term additional cardiac output for the duration of the procedure and for several hours afterward. In a retrospective single-center study, Flaherty and colleagues[12] reviewed 230 matched cases of patients undergoing PCI supported with the Impella 2.5 device, with a significantly lower incidence of CI-AKI (5.2% vs 27.8%; OR, 0.13; 95% confidence interval, 0.09–0.31; $P<.001$). These data are preliminary, however, and likely to have unmeasured confounders. Larger randomized trials are required to firmly answer this question.

Contrast volume and the development of contrast-induced acute kidney injury

There is a clear correlation between the volume of contrast media and the risk of developing CI-AKI. A recent large registry of 182,196 patients undergoing PCI demonstrated an observational association between a reduction in contrast volumes and the development of AKI.[13] Data from the CathPCI registry, reflecting more than 1.3 million patients, revealed a consistent association with contrast volume and the development of AKI (OR, 1.42 per incremental 7 mL increase in contrast volume, adjusted for patient characteristics and AKI risk).[14] The threshold of volume at which CI-AKI develops depends multiple patient factors, captured with predictive risk scores such as the Mehran or Gurm score. Laskey and colleagues[15] demonstrated that a ratio of contrast volume to creatinine clearance of greater than 3.7 was strongly associated with CI-AKI, and this value is noted in the European Society of Cardiology and Society for Cardiovascular Angiography and Interventions guidelines for coronary intervention in regard to delaying a staged procedure.

Contrast Volume Minimization

Several approaches can conceptually be used to limit the volume of contrast delivered to a patient. Most simply, the volume of contrast delivered during each injection can be minimized, provided adequate coronary visualization is obtained. Indeed, several reports describing coronary interventions with volumes of less than 20 mL (without additional imaging) have been reported. In an alternate strategy, the volume of radiographic contrast received by a patient can be limited by decreasing coronary reflux. Although some reflux is necessary for adequate visualization of the coronary ostia, most of the refluxed dye provides no angiographic benefit. A series of devices designed to minimize contrast reflux by optimizing the delivery profile have been developed by Osprey Medical (Minnetonka, MN). The first-generation AVERT device was a manually adjusted system in which excess contrast was returned to a reservoir chamber that exists between the injection syringe and the manifold by balancing the resistance between the contrast delivery path and that of the resistance to contrast entry into the collection chamber. A study of 587 patients undergoing coronary angiography demonstrated a 16% decrease in contrast volume (with greater relative decreases in procedures involving ≥3 lesions), although there was no reduction in rates of CI-AKI.[16] A second generation of this approach (DyeVert, Osprey Medical) has been developed in which manual resistance adjustment is not required. A study of 114 patients with a baseline glomerular filtration rate of 20 to 60 mL/min/1.73 m^2 using the DyeVert system showed a decrease in delivered contrast volume of 40%, with no loss of angiographic quality, although this was a single-arm observational study and underpowered to detect a difference in the development of CI-AKI.[17] The DyeMINISH global patient registry is currently enrolling up to 10,000 patients to measure real-world outcomes, expected to complete in late 2023.

Coronary Sinus Contrast Removal

Because the contrast media is cleared from the myocardium via the coronary sinus, devices have been developed to directly remove contrast media after each intracoronary injection, before the exposure to the kidneys. In a study by Duffy and colleagues[18] of the CI-AKICOR Contrast Removal System, 26 patients with impaired renal function underwent coronary sinus cannulation before angiography. Seventy-five percent of patients were successfully cannulated, with an average of 169 ± 15 mL withdrawn, with spectroscopy demonstrating recapture of around one-third of the delivered contrast. The matched comparator group had a statistically significant decrease in the estimated glomerular filtration rate (−2.5 ± 0.5 mL/min), with no significant change in the coronary sinus cannulation group; however, there was a greater decrease in hemoglobin in those undergoing intervention.

Automated Contrast Injection

Automated systems for contrast injectors have been demonstrated to significantly decrease contrast volume delivery. A meta-analysis from Minsinger and colleagues[19] of 79,694 patients across 10 studies demonstrated a decrease in volume of 45 mL per case, with a decrease in the incidence of CI-AKI of 15%. Benefits were seen across both diagnostic angiography and PCI, and across various catheter diameters from 4F to 6F. An ultra-low contrast delivery technique has also been described,[20] involving reprogramming over the automated injector after the first injection tailored to an individual contrast spillover profile and coronary size. The ultra-low contrast delivery algorithm resulted in a significantly lower contrast volume (24 ± 20 mL vs 48 ± 31 mL; P<.01). Importantly, the use of the ultra-low contrast delivery technique shortened the procedure time. A longer term study powered for clinical events including CI-AKI is required to evaluate the benefit of this technique.

Renal Replacement Therapy

Hemodialysis is an effective method for contrast removal, with up to 80% of contrast removed over a 4-hour period. Blood flow, membrane surface area, molecular size, transmembrane pressure, and dialysis time are all key determinants of effectiveness. Despite the removal of contrast, however, renal replacement therapies are invasive and may induce inflammation, coagulation, and hypotension, thereby worsening renal function.

Conversely, the relatively gentler approach of hemofiltration may offer benefit. A study of 114 patients with chronic kidney disease (creatinine of >2 mg/dL) undergoing coronary angiography were randomized to hemofiltration or hydration by Marenzi and colleagues,[21] with a marked decrease in the development of CI-AKI (defined as an increase in creatinine of >25% from baseline), as well as in both short- and long-term mortality. A follow-up study determined that hemofiltration performed before intervention was more useful than when initiated afterward; however, renal replacement therapy is not currently guideline recommended to prevent CI-AKI.

Prevention of Thromboembolism

Although not the primary mechanism of CI-AKI, thromboembolism is an important consideration when performing coronary and structural procedures because the femoral approach may lead to more frequent atheroemboli to the renal circulation. The AKI-MATRIX study was a substudy of the MATRIX-Access study, evaluating 8210 patients with acute coronary syndromes. AKI was slightly less frequent in patients undergoing angiography from the radial approach compared with femoral cases (OR, 0.87; 95% confidence interval, 0.77–0.98; $P = .018$).[22]

Zero and ultra-low contrast percutaneous coronary intervention

If contrast is not used for percutaneous intervention, then contrast-induced kidney injury cannot occur. The concept of zero and ultra-low contrast PCI has been of increasing interest over the past decade with the rise of advanced intracoronary imaging techniques such as intravascular ultrasound examination and optical coherence tomography. The MOZART trial[23] randomized 83 patients to either angiography guided PCI or intravascular ultrasound examination–guided PCI, with a reduction in contrast volume by 45 mL (65 mL vs 20 mL) in the latter group. There was no significant difference in outcomes out to 4 months; however, the overall study group was underpowered to detect this difference. Optical coherence tomography relies on the vessel lumen being flushed to clear blood to improve image quality; although traditionally done with contrast media, dextran-based optical coherence tomography has been successfully performed with little loss in image quality.[24] Dextran is potentially nephrotoxic in large volumes, however, with further evaluation required in larger trials.

Imaging system technology

Stent enhancement technologies such as StentBoost (Philips, Best, the Netherlands) or ClearStent (Siemens Healthcare, Erlangen, Germany) can permit positioning of postdilation balloons without additional contrast. More recently, the Dynamic Coronary Roadmap (Philips) provide the clinician with real-time live navigational guidance with an overlaid coronary image, further reducing the need for additional contrast test shots. Biplane imaging can also provide multiple views with a single injection, decreasing contrast volume further.

Tracking contrast use

Contrast volume should be recorded with each case and is considered a key performance metric for catheter laboratory performance. The DyeVert system tracks contrast volume accurately and automatically; cost-effective systems that provide similar information to clinicians during a case may result in modification during the procedure to contrast delivery, however this has not been evaluated specifically in a catheter laboratory setting, although benefits have been seen in the radiology setting.

SUMMARY

CI-AKI is not uncommon after coronary angiography, and a limited number of effective pharmacologic agents exist for prevention. Device-based therapies thus far have mainly shown benefit by either guiding intravenous hydration or decreasing contrast administration, with several novel devices on the horizon. Large-scale randomized clinical trials are required to show benefit on hard clinical end points to provide clinicians with support in the prevention of CI-AKI.

ACKNOWLEDGMENTS

S. Nanayakkara is supported by a scholarship from the National Heart Foundation of Australia (101116) and the Baker Bright Sparks program. D.M. Kaye is supported by a Fellowship from the National Health and Medical Research Council of Australia. The Baker Institute is supported in part by the Victorian Government's OIS Program.

DISCLOSURE

D.M. Kaye is the co-founder of Osprey Medical.

REFERENCES

1. Rear R, Bell RM, Hausenloy DJ. Contrast-induced nephropathy following angiography and cardiac interventions. Heart 2016;102(8):638–48.
2. Almendarez M, Gurm HS, Mariani J, et al. Procedural strategies to reduce the incidence of contrast-induced acute kidney injury during percutaneous coronary intervention. JACC Cardiovasc Interv 2019;12(19):1877–88.
3. Er F, Nia AM, Dopp H, et al. Ischemic preconditioning for prevention of contrast medium–induced nephropathy: randomized pilot renpro trial (renal protection trial). Circulation 2012;126(3):296–303.
4. Deftereos S, Giannopoulos G, Tzalamouras V, et al. Renoprotective effect of remote ischemic postconditioning by intermittent balloon inflations in patients undergoing percutaneous coronary intervention. J Am Coll Cardiol 2013;61(19):1949–55.
5. Weisz G, Filby SJ, Cohen MG, et al. Safety and performance of targeted renal therapy: the Be-RITe! Registry. J Endovasc Ther 2009;16(1):1–12.
6. Brar SS, Aharonian V, Mansukhani P, et al. Haemodynamic-guided fluid administration for the prevention of contrast-induced acute kidney injury: the POSEIDON randomised controlled trial. Lancet 2014;383(9931):1814–23.
7. Solomon R, Werner C, Mann D, et al. Effects of saline, mannitol, and furosemide on acute decreases in renal function induced by radiocontrast agents. N Engl J Med 1994;331(21):1416–20.
8. Briguori C, D'Amore C, De Micco F, et al. Renal insufficiency following contrast media administration trial III: Urine flow rate-guided versus left-ventricular end-diastolic pressure-guided hydration in high-risk patients for contrast-induced acute kidney injury. Rationale and design. Catheter Cardiovasc Interv 2020;95(5):895–903.
9. Mehran R, Aymong ED, Nikolsky E, et al. A simple risk score for prediction of contrast-induced nephropathy after percutaneous coronary intervention: development and initial validation. J Am Coll Cardiol 2004;44(7):1393–9.
10. Gurm HS, Seth M, Kooiman J, et al. A novel tool for reliable and accurate prediction of renal complications in patients undergoing percutaneous coronary intervention. J Am Coll Cardiol 2013;61(22):2242–8.
11. Maioli M, Toso A, Leoncini M, et al. Bioimpedance-guided hydration for the prevention of contrast-induced kidney Injury. J Am Coll Cardiol 2018;71(25):2880–9.
12. Flaherty MP, Pant S, Patel SV, et al. Hemodynamic support with a microaxial percutaneous left ventricular assist device (impella) protects against acute kidney injury in patients undergoing high-risk percutaneous coronary intervention. Circ Res 2017;120(4):692–700.
13. Gurm HS, Seth M, Dixon S, et al. Trends in contrast volume use and incidence of acute kidney injury in patients undergoing percutaneous coronary intervention. JACC Cardiovasc Interv 2018;11(5):509–11.
14. Amin AP, Bach RG, Caruso ML, et al. Association of variation in contrast volume with acute kidney injury in patients undergoing percutaneous coronary intervention. JAMA Cardiol 2017;2(9):1007–12.
15. Laskey WK, Jenkins C, Selzer F, et al. Volume-to-creatinine clearance ratio: a pharmacokinetically based risk factor for prediction of early creatinine increase after percutaneous coronary intervention. J Am Coll Cardiol 2007;50(7):584–90.
16. Mehran R, Faggioni M, Chandrasekhar J, et al. Effect of a contrast modulation system on contrast media use and the rate of acute kidney injury after coronary angiography. JACC Cardiovasc Interv 2018;11(16):1601–10.
17. Gurm HS, Mavromatis K, Bertolet B, et al. Minimizing radiographic contrast administration during coronary angiography using a novel contrast reduction system: a multicenter observational study of the DyeVert™ plus contrast reduction system. Catheter Cardiovasc Interv 2019;93(7):1228–35.
18. Duffy SJ, Ruygrok P, Juergens CP, et al. Removal of contrast media from the coronary sinus attenuates renal injury after coronary angiography and intervention. J Am Coll Cardiol 2010;56(6):525–6.
19. Minsinger KD, Kassis HM, Block CA, et al. Meta-analysis of the effect of automated contrast injection devices versus manual injection and contrast volume on risk of contrast induced nephropathy. Am J Cardiol 2014;113(1):49–53.
20. Stys A, Gedela M, Bhatnagar U, et al. A prospective study of contrast preservation using ultra-low contrast delivery technique versus standard automated contrast injector system in coronary procedures. Indian Heart J 2019;71(4):297–302.
21. Marenzi G, Marana I, Lauri G, et al. The prevention of radiocontrast-agent-induced nephropathy by hemofiltration. N Engl J Med 2003;349(14):1333–40.

22. Andò G, Cortese B, Russo F, et al. Acute kidney injury after radial or femoral access for invasive acute coronary syndrome management: AKI-MA-TRIX. J Am Coll Cardiol 2017. https://doi.org/10.1016/j.jacc.2017.02.070.

23. Mariani J, Guedes C, Soares P, et al. Intravascular ultrasound guidance to minimize the use of iodine contrast in percutaneous coronary intervention: the MOZART (Minimizing cOntrast utiliZation With IVUS Guidance in coRonary angioplasTy) randomized controlled trial. JACC Cardiovasc Interv 2014; 7(11):1287–93.

24. Azzalini L, Laricchia A, Regazzoli D, et al. Ultra-low contrast percutaneous coronary intervention to minimize the risk for contrast-induced acute kidney injury in patients with severe chronic kidney disease. J Invasive Cardiol 2019;31(6): 176–82.

A Practical Approach to Preventing Renal Complications in the Catheterization Laboratory

Devika Aggarwal, MD[a], Hitinder S. Gurm, MD[b],*

KEYWORDS
• Contrast-induced acute kidney injury • Ultra-low contrast volume
• Renal function-based contrast dosing

KEY POINTS
• Implementation of preventive strategies key to reducing contast-induced acute kidney injury.
• Identify at-risk patients using risk prediction models, such as the BMC2 risk prediction tool, to target preventive strategies effectively.
• Adopt a hydration protocol using a combination of oral and intravenous hydration.
• Limit contrast volume to less than 2-3 times the eGFR, and attempt to use ultra-low contrast volume in highest-risk patients.

INTRODUCTION

Contrast-induced acute kidney injury (CI-AKI) is believed to result from the direct toxicity of contrast media on tubular epithelial cells as well as indirect hypoxic injury.[1–4] In a nationwide study examining nearly 1 million consecutive percutaneous coronary interventions (PCIs), CI-AKI was reported in 7.1% of patients, with 0.3% patients developing a new need for dialysis.[5] Development of CI-AKI, in turn, is associated with increased mortality, recurrent myocardial infarction (MI), sustained reduction in kidney function, and longer hospital stay.[5–12] With no specific treatment for CI-AKI, implementation of effective preventive strategies is central to reducing the burden of CI-AKI.

Over the past 2 decades, many studies have investigated different, and at times innovative methods for preventing CI-AKI, with equivocal results. The risk of CI-AKI is directly but nonlinearly associated with the volume of contrast media reaching the distal renal tubule, and strategies that reduce the volume and concentration of contrast in the renal tubule appear to reduce the incidence of CI-AKI. Effective preventive strategies for reducing the risk of CI-AKI are based on key elementary principles: identification of high-risk patients, intravascular volume expansion, pharmaceutical agents, and minimization of contrast media. In this review, we discuss the rationale and efficacy of the different methods and suggest a practical approach to prevent CI-AKI.

IDENTIFYING HIGH-RISK PATIENTS

As compared with the general population, the incidence of CI-AKI after PCI is significantly greater in high-risk patients. Recognizing the risk factors and targeting preventive strategies to high-risk patients can reduce the occurrence of CI-AKI in a feasible and cost-effective manner. Tsai and colleagues[5] reported severe preexisting chronic kidney disease (CKD), ST-segment elevation MI presentation, and cardiogenic

[a] Department of Internal Medicine, Beaumont Hospital-Royal Oak, 3601 W 13 Mile Road, Royal Oak, MI 48073, USA; [b] Department of Internal Medicine, Division of Cardiovascular Medicine, University of Michigan, 2A 192F, 1500 East Medical Center Drive, Ann Arbor, MI 48109-5853, USA
* Corresponding author.
E-mail address: hgurm@med.umich.edu

Intervent Cardiol Clin 9 (2020) 403–407
https://doi.org/10.1016/j.iccl.2020.02.011
2211-7458/20/© 2020 Elsevier Inc. All rights reserved.

shock as the strongest predictors of CI-AKI. Diabetes and anemia not only increase the susceptibility in patients with CKD but also are independently associated with an increase in CI-AKI.[13–16]

Several risk prediction models have been proposed for the identification of at-risk patients. The most commonly used scores, described by Mehran and colleagues[15] and Bartholomew and colleagues,[7] include procedural variables, such as contrast volume, limiting their utility. Prediction tools considering only preprocedural variables are preferable, as they can help in making informed patient-level decisions and target preventive strategies to patients at high risk. The tools proposed by Tsai and colleagues,[17] Brown and colleagues,[18] and Gurm and colleagues[19] are derived from large cohorts, have good discriminative power, and can be used in predicting the risk of CI-AKI before PCI. The BMC2 risk prediction tool has the best discrimination of the currently available risk models, is available as a downloadable app as well as a Web-based calculator, and is our preferred tool.[19]

HYDRATION

Decreasing the concentration of contrast media reaching the renal tubules by dilution is the key rationale for the benefit of fluid administration for prevention of CI-AKI.[20] Although the choice of fluid has been debated exhaustively, multiple large studies and meta-analyses have reported no benefit of sodium bicarbonate over isotonic sodium chloride.[21–23] The American College of Cardiology Foundation (ACCF)/American Heart Association (AHA)/Society for Cardiovascular Angiography and Interventions (SCAI) guidelines assign a Class I (Level of Evidence: B) for adequate preparatory hydration for patients undergoing cardiac catheterization.[24] These recommendations were challenged by the recent AMACING (A MAastricht Contrast-Induced Nephropathy Guideline) trial, which demonstrated that no prophylaxis was noninferior to periprocedural hydration in the prevention of CI-AKI.[25] However, this study had a modest size and a very low event rate. Because of these limitations, it would be premature to dismiss the role of fluid administration in the prevention of CI-AKI until more corroborative data are available.

Modifying the traditional NPO or nil per ora orders and permitting water intake helps in maintaining a euvolemic state, is cost-effective, and improves patient satisfaction.[26] Several small studies have reported no significant difference in the incidence of CI-AKI with oral water intake or parenteral fluids, as long as a certain volume of water has been specified.[27] With regard to the duration and rate of volume expansion, there are no definitive recommendations. The POSEIDON (Prevention of Contrast Renal Injury with Different Hydration Strategies) trial demonstrated that in comparison with standard infusion protocols (1.5 mL/kg), left ventricular end-diastolic pressure–guided parenteral hydration was well tolerated and had a significantly lower rate of CI-AKI.[28] Another strategy using urine flow rate as a guide to parenteral hydration has shown promising results in preventing CI-AKI in high-risk patients.[29,30] However, this usually requires the use of a urinary catheter and is not ideal for routine practice. Because volume expansion remains the cornerstone of CI-AKI prevention, catheterization laboratories should adopt a practical hydration protocol using a combination of oral and intravenous fluids that can be seamlessly adopted in routine practice (Fig. 1).

PHARMACOLOGICAL AGENTS

Pharmacologic prophylaxis has been an area of intense focus in the field of CI-AKI. N-acetylcysteine, one of the most researched agents, has not been shown to prevent CI-AKI, or other clinically relevant endpoints, and its use has largely been abandoned globally.[23,31]

Statins are the primary class of drugs currently used for the prevention of CI-AKI. In the randomized PRATO-ACS (Protective Effect of Rosuvastatin and Antiplatelet Therapy On contrast-induced acute kidney injury and myocardial damage in patients with Acute Coronary Syndrome) trial that included statin-naïve patients with non-ST-segment elevation MI, the incidence of CI-AKI was significantly lower in patients receiving high-dose rosuvastatin as compared with the control group.[32] This acute nephroprotective effect of statins has been ascribed to their anti-inflammatory, antioxidant, and antithrombotic properties. Additional trials and meta-analyses have reported mixed results, with some advocating for and some against pretreatment with statins.[33,34] This ambiguity extends to recommendations from professional societies. Although the European Society of Cardiology gives a Class IIa (Level of Evidence: A) recommendation for pretreatment with high-dose statins in patients with moderate-severe CKD, the ACCF/AHA/SCAI guidelines have no mention of statins in the prevention of CI-AKI.[35] Regardless, statins are a cornerstone

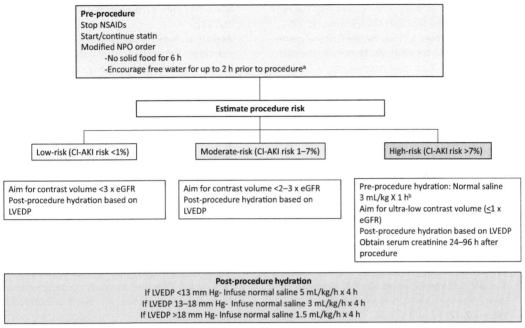

Fig. 1. Approach to prevention of contrast-induced acute kidney injury. LVEDP, left ventricular end-diastolic pressure; NSAIDs, nonsteroidal anti-inflammatory drugs. [a]Avoid oral prehydration in patients with gastroparesis, those undergoing procedures under general anesthesia, and those with active heart failure. [b]Avoid intravenous prehydration in patients with severe valve disease, and/or known congestive heart failure.

drug in contemporary practice and are indicated for coronary artery disease and should be standard therapy in patients undergoing PCI.

CONTRAST MINIMIZATION

The volume of contrast administered is considered the strongest modifiable procedural factor associated with CI-AKI and new need for dialysis.[36,37] Limiting the volume of contrast to less than 3, and preferably 2 times the baseline estimated glomerular filtration rate (eGFR) is associated with a significantly lower risk of CI-AKI.[38,39] Furthermore, patients with the highest risk of CI-AKI may benefit from the use of "ultra-low" contrast volume (less than or equal to the eGFR).[40,41] This strategy is growing in practice and is especially effective in high-risk patients.

OTHER PREVENTIVE STRATEGIES

A careful review of the patient's medications and withdrawal of potentially nephrotoxic agents, like nonsteroidal anti-inflammatory drugs, during the periprocedural period is advised.[42] However, there is insufficient evidence regarding the interruption of diuretics, angiotensin-converting enzyme inhibitors, and angiotensin receptor blockers. Although many catheterization laboratories routinely hold metformin before

catheterization for fear of lactic acidosis secondary to CI-AKI, this precautionary approach has never been formally validated in a randomized setting. An alternative approach of stopping metformin in case of declining renal function is a reasonable recommendation by the European Society of Cardiology.[35] Despite removing contrast media, prophylactic renal replacement therapy has not shown benefit in reducing CI-AKI and is not routinely recommended.[43]

In conclusion, CI-AKI is an infrequent but consequential complication of invasive cardiovascular procedures, with limited effective options for prevention. A combination of intravascular volume expansion and contrast minimization, the 2 main strategies backed by data, can be easily implemented. We suggest one such approach in **Fig. 1**. Standard adoption of this or similar processes in the catheterization laboratory can significantly reduce the occurrence of CI-AKI.[44]

REFERENCES

1. Katzberg RW. Contrast medium-induced nephrotoxicity: which pathway? Radiology 2005. https://doi.org/10.1148/radiol.2353041865.
2. Heyman SN, Rosen S, Brezis M. Radiocontrast nephropathy: a paradigm for the synergism between

toxic and hypoxic insults in the kidney. Exp Nephrol 1994. https://doi.org/10.1148/radiology.195.1.82.

3. Heyman SN, Rosen S, Rosenberger C. Renal parenchymal hypoxia, hypoxia adaptation, and the pathogenesis of radiocontrast nephropathy. Clin J Am Soc Nephrol 2008. https://doi.org/10.2215/CJN.02600607.

4. Haller C, Hizoh I. The cytotoxicity of iodinated radiocontrast agents on renal cells in vitro. Invest Radiol 2004. https://doi.org/10.1097/01.rli.0000113776.87762.49.

5. Tsai TT, Patel UD, Chang TI, et al. Contemporary incidence, predictors, and outcomes of acute kidney injury in patients undergoing percutaneous coronary interventions: insights from the NCDR cath-PCI registry. JACC Cardiovasc Interv 2014. https://doi.org/10.1016/j.jcin.2013.06.016.

6. Kooiman J, Seth M, Nallamothu BK, et al. Association between acute kidney injury and in-hospital mortality in patients undergoing percutaneous coronary interventions. Circ Cardiovasc Interv 2015; 8(6):e002212.

7. Bartholomew BA, Harjai KJ, Dukkipati S, et al. Impact of nephropathy after percutaneous coronary intervention and a method for risk stratification. Am J Cardiol 2004;93(12):1515–9.

8. Lindsay J, Apple S, Pinnow EE, et al. Percutaneous coronary intervention-associated nephropathy foreshadows increased risk of late adverse events in patients with normal baseline serum creatinine. Catheter Cardiovasc Interv 2003;59(3):338–43.

9. Dangas G, Iakovou I, Nikolsky E, et al. Contrast-induced nephropathy after percutaneous coronary interventions in relation to chronic kidney disease and hemodynamic variables. Am J Cardiol 2005; 95(1):13–9.

10. James MT, Samuel SM, Manning MA, et al. Contrast-induced acute kidney injury and risk of adverse clinical outcomes after coronary angiography: a systematic review and meta-analysis. Circ Cardiovasc Interv 2013;6(1):37–43.

11. James MT, Ghali WA, Tonelli M, et al. Acute kidney injury following coronary angiography is associated with a long-term decline in kidney function. Kidney Int 2010;78(8):803–9.

12. Marenzi G, Lauri G, Assanelli E, et al. Contrast-induced nephropathy in patients undergoing primary angioplasty for acute myocardial infarction. J Am Coll Cardiol 2004;44(9):1780–5.

13. Rudnick MR, Goldfarb S, Wexler L, et al. Nephrotoxicity of ionic and nonionic contrast media in 1196 patients: a randomized trial. Kidney Int 1995. https://doi.org/10.1038/ki.1995.32.

14. McCullough PA, Wolyn R, Rocher LL, et al. Acute renal failure after coronary intervention: incidence, risk factors, and relationship to mortality. Am J Med 1997. https://doi.org/10.1016/S0002-9343(97)00150-2.

15. Mehran R, Aymong ED, Nikolsky E, et al. A simple risk score for prediction of contrast-induced nephropathy after percutaneous coronary intervention: development and initial validation. J Am Coll Cardiol 2004. https://doi.org/10.1016/j.jacc.2004.06.068.

16. Nikolsky E, Mehran R, Lasic Z, et al. Low hematocrit predicts contrast-induced nephropathy after percutaneous coronary interventions. Kidney Int 2005. https://doi.org/10.1111/j.1523-1755.2005.67131.x.

17. Tsai TT, Patel UD, Chang TI, et al. Validated contemporary risk model of acute kidney injury in patients undergoing percutaneous coronary interventions: Insights from the National Cardiovascular Data Registry Cath-PCI registry. J Am Heart Assoc 2014. https://doi.org/10.1161/JAHA.114.001380.

18. Brown JR, DeVries JT, Piper WD, et al. Serious renal dysfunction after percutaneous coronary interventions can be predicted. Am Heart J 2008;155(2):260–6.

19. Gurm HS, Seth M, Kooiman J, et al. A novel tool for reliable and accurate prediction of renal complications in patients undergoing percutaneous coronary intervention. J Am Coll Cardiol 2013;61(22):2242–8.

20. Rojkovskiy I, Solomon R. Intravenous and oral hydration: approaches, principles, and differing regimens. Interv Cardiol Clin 2014;3(3):393–404.

21. Brar SS. Sodium bicarbonate vs sodium chloride for the prevention of contrast medium–induced nephropathy in patients undergoing coronary angiography: a randomized trial. JAMA 2008;300(9):1038.

22. Solomon R, Gordon P, Manoukian SV, et al. Randomized trial of bicarbonate or saline study for the prevention of contrast-induced nephropathy in patients with CKD. Clin J Am Soc Nephrol 2015;10(9):1519–24.

23. Weisbord SD, Gallagher M, Jneid H, et al. Outcomes after angiography with sodium bicarbonate and acetylcysteine. N Engl J Med 2018;378(7):603–14.

24. Levine GN, Bates ER, Blankenship JC, et al. 2011 ACCF/AHA/SCAI guideline for percutaneous coronary intervention: a report of the American College of Cardiology Foundation/American Heart Association Task Force on Practice Guidelines and the Society for Cardiovascular Angiography and Interventions. Circulation 2011;124(23):e574–651.

25. Nijssen EC, Rennenberg RJ, Nelemans PJ, et al. Prophylactic hydration to protect renal function from intravascular iodinated contrast material in patients at high risk of contrast-induced nephropathy (AMACING): a prospective, randomised, phase 3, controlled, open-label, non-inferiority trial. Lancet 2017;389(10076):1312–22.

26. Bittl JA. A proposal to reduce contrast nephropathy: eliminate the NPO order. Catheter Cardiovasc Interv 2014;83(6):913–4.

27. Agarwal SK, Mohareb S, Patel A, et al. Systematic oral hydration with water is similar to parenteral hydration for prevention of contrast-induced nephropathy: an updated meta-analysis of randomised clinical data. Open Heart 2015;2(1):e000317.

28. Brar SS, Aharonian V, Mansukhani P, et al. Haemodynamic-guided fluid administration for the prevention of contrast-induced acute kidney injury: the POSEIDON randomised controlled trial. Lancet 2014;383(9931):1814–23.

29. Briguori C, Visconti G, Focaccio A, et al. Renal insufficiency after contrast media administration trial II (REMEDIAL II): renalGuard System in high-risk patients for contrast-induced acute kidney injury. Circulation 2011;124(11):1260–9.

30. Marenzi G, Ferrari C, Marana I, et al. Prevention of contrast nephropathy by furosemide with matched hydration: the MYTHOS (Induced Diuresis With Matched Hydration Compared to Standard Hydration for Contrast Induced Nephropathy Prevention) trial. JACC Cardiovasc Interv 2012;5(1):90–7.

31. ACT Investigators. Acetylcysteine for prevention of renal outcomes in patients undergoing coronary and peripheral vascular angiography: main results from the randomized Acetylcysteine for Contrast-induced nephropathy Trial (ACT). Circulation 2011;124(11):1250–9.

32. Leoncini M, Toso A, Maioli M, et al. Early high-dose rosuvastatin for contrast-induced nephropathy prevention in acute coronary syndrome: results from the PRATO-ACS Study (Protective Effect of Rosuvastatin and Antiplatelet Therapy On Contrast-Induced Acute Kidney Injury and Myocardial Damage in Patients With Acute Coronary Syndrome). J Am Coll Cardiol 2014;63(1):71–9.

33. Jo S-H, Koo B-K, Park J-S, et al. Prevention of radiocontrast medium-induced nephropathy using short-term high-dose simvastatin in patients with renal insufficiency undergoing coronary angiography (PROMISS) trial—a randomized controlled study. Am Heart J 2008;155(3):499.e1-8.

34. Giacoppo D, Gargiulo G, Buccheri S, et al. Preventive strategies for contrast-induced acute kidney injury in patients undergoing percutaneous coronary procedures: evidence from a hierarchical bayesian network meta-analysis of 124 trials and 28 240 patients. Circ Cardiovasc Interv 2017;10(5).

35. Neumann F-J, Sousa-Uva M, Ahlsson A, et al. 2018 ESC/EACTS guidelines on myocardial revascularization. Eur Heart J 2019;40(2):87–165.

36. Marenzi G. Contrast volume during primary percutaneous coronary intervention and subsequent contrast-induced nephropathy and mortality. Ann Intern Med 2009;150(3):170.

37. Freeman RV, O'Donnell M, Share D, et al. Nephropathy requiring dialysis after percutaneous coronary intervention and the critical role of an adjusted contrast dose. Am J Cardiol 2002;90(10):1068–73.

38. Gurm HS, Dixon SR, Smith DE, et al. Renal function-based contrast dosing to define safe limits of radiographic contrast media in patients undergoing percutaneous coronary interventions. J Am Coll Cardiol 2011. https://doi.org/10.1016/j.jacc.2011.05.023.

39. Andò G, De Gregorio C, Morabito G, et al. Renal function-adjusted contrast volume redefines the baseline estimation of contrast-induced acute kidney injury risk in patients undergoing primary percutaneous coronary intervention. Circ Cardiovasc Interv 2014. https://doi.org/10.1161/CIRCINTERVENTIONS.114.001545.

40. Kane GC, Doyle BJ, Lerman A, et al. Ultra-low contrast volumes reduce rates of contrast-induced nephropathy in patients with chronic kidney disease undergoing coronary angiography. J Am Coll Cardiol 2008. https://doi.org/10.1016/j.jacc.2007.09.019.

41. Gurm HS, Seth M, Dixon SR, et al. Contemporary use of and outcomes associated with ultra-low contrast volume in patients undergoing percutaneous coronary interventions. Catheter Cardiovasc Interv 2019. https://doi.org/10.1002/ccd.27819.

42. McCullough PA. Contrast-induced acute kidney injury. J Am Coll Cardiol 2008;51(15):1419–28.

43. Cruz DN, Goh CY, Marenzi G, et al. Renal replacement therapies for prevention of radiocontrast-induced nephropathy: a systematic review. Am J Med 2012;125(1):66–78.e3.

44. Gurm HS, Seth M, Dixon S, et al. Trends in contrast volume use and incidence of acute kidney injury in patients undergoing percutaneous coronary intervention: insights from blue cross blue shield of michigan cardiovascular collaborative (BMC2). JACC Cardiovasc Interv 2018;11(5):509–11.